Ayurveda

*

The Science of

Traditional
Indian Medicine

*

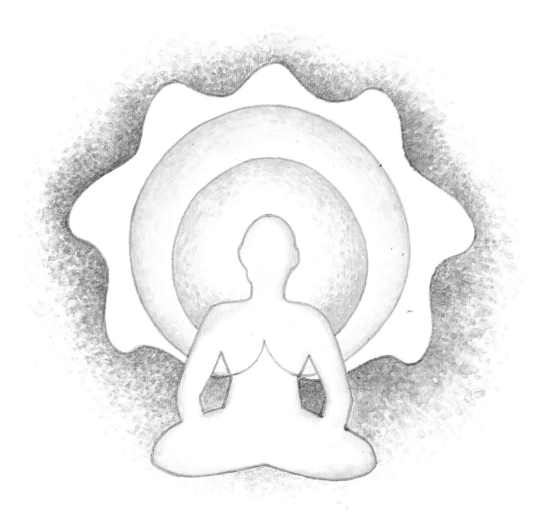

Meditation gives the mind peace which keeps the body healthy and the spirit calm.
Ayurveda is a holistic form of medicine which emphasises the balance of
the body-mind-spirit complex.

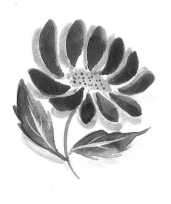
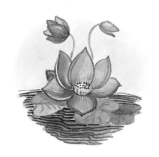
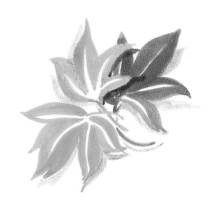

Ayurveda

*

The Science of
Traditional
Indian Medicine

*

VAIDYA BHAGWAN DASH
SUHASINI RAMASWAMY

Lustre Press
Roli Books

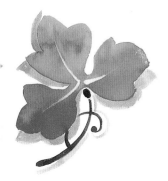
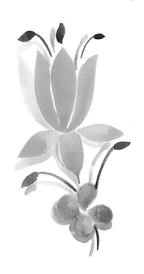

© **Lustre Press Pvt. Ltd. 1998**

Third impression 2002
Lustre Press Pvt. Ltd.
M-75, GK II Market
New Delhi-110 048, INDIA
Tel: (011) 6442271, 6462782, 6460886
Fax: (011) 6467185
E-mail: roli@vsnl.com
Website: rolibooks.com

ISBN: 81-7436-044-1

Authors:

Vaidya Bhagwan Dash
Suhasini Ramaswamy

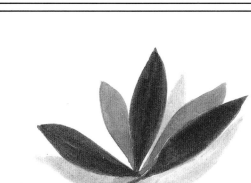

Illustrations:

A. V. Prasanth

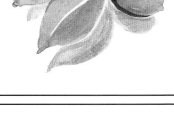
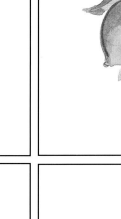

Printed and bound by

Star Standard Industries Pte. Ltd.,
Singapore

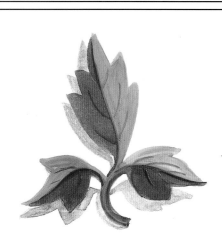

Conceived & Designed
at
ROLI CAD CENTRE

The Meaning
of Ayurveda

7

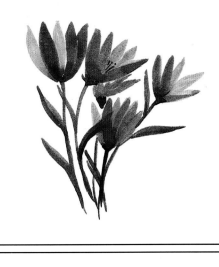

The Natural Body
Constitution

13

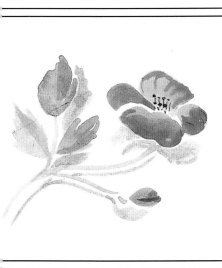

Causes and Diagnosis
of Diseases

25

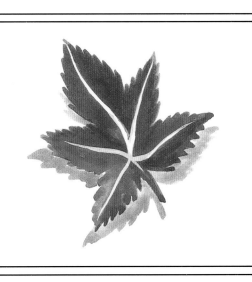

Treatment of
Diseases

33

Measures for
Good Health

70

Glossary

81

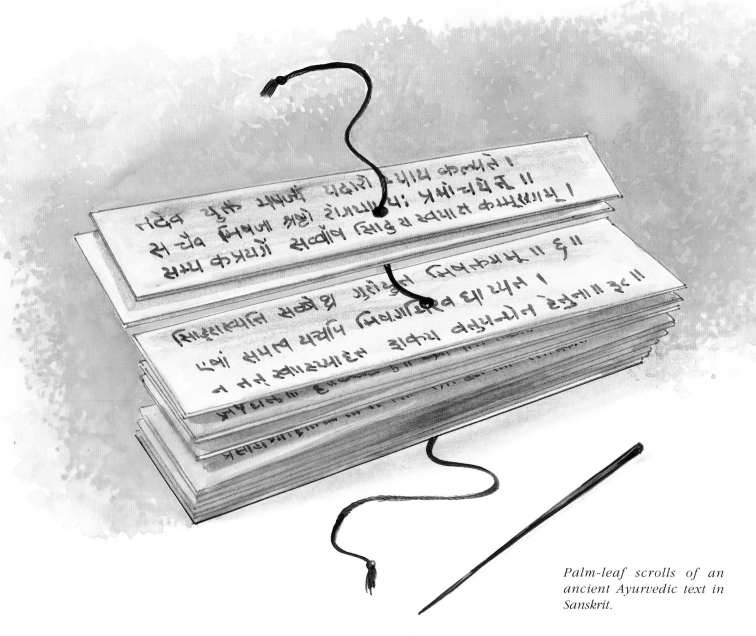

Palm-leaf scrolls of an ancient Ayurvedic text in Sanskrit.

The Meaning of Ayurveda

———— ✳ ————

Traditional systems of medicine like Ayurveda have become popular in recent years. This is part of the renewed interest in ethnic cultures the world over, in their lifestyles and religious beliefs. Medicine may be seen as a living component of an unbroken tradition stretching back to several centuries. In India and her neighbours like Nepal, Sri Lanka, Bangladesh and Pakistan, such systems have long been in existence and studied scientifically and codified, with written texts that have been preserved through the ages. Passed on from one generation to another, they have

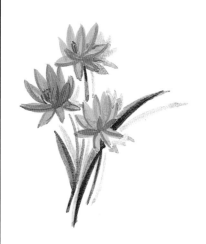

Ayurveda is that which deals with good, bad, happy and unhappy life, its promoters and non-promoters, measurements and nature.

. . . Charaka (Tr. P.V. Sarma)

stood the test of time. Of the many systems, Ayurveda is perhaps the best known and most widely prevalent.

These systems are unique in that they are deeply rooted in traditional cultures and draw upon their wisdom, knowledge and experience. But at the same time, because they emanate from man's interaction with the environment or the macrocosm, they are applicable universally. They may be termed as alternative systems of medicine only in relation to modern Western medicine. Ayurveda and other such systems are both supplementary and complementary to modern medicine in helping to provide good health to humanity.

Despite the advances in modern medicine, there are many drugs which often cause toxic side-effects. Painkillers and palliative measures offer only temporary relief. This has influenced the need for other kinds of treatment. A visible shift is also evident today from the over specialisation which characterizes modern medical science to a more holistic viewpoint in the treatment of diseases. Holistic medicine as in Ayurveda, deals with the body-mind-spirit complex. More than the specific disease, it is the patient who is sought to be treated.

Good health thus becomes a whole way of life which may be achieved by adopting certain general principles of behaviour and following certain regimens. Diseases may not only be cured but in fact may be prevented by observing these rules.

Ayurveda also draws upon other traditional systems of medicine like naturopathy, Tibetan Buddhist medicine and Unani tibb (Graeco-Arabic medicine) since in theory and practice there is a high degree of commonality among them. Practitioners of one system freely use the medicinal products of the other as they are all products of nature.

The word Ayurveda is made up of two Sanskrit words *ayur* and *veda* meaning 'life' and 'knowledge' respectively. Taken together they mean the 'science of life'; in a more limited sense, the term is used to imply the science of medicine.

The origins of Ayurveda are shrouded in antiquity. Legend says that Brahma the Creator, a part of the Hindu holy trinity of gods, first perceived it and taught it to his son, Daksha-Prajapati. Subsequently, Lord Dhanwantari, the god of healing and the teacher of the medical sciences passed it on to the prominent Hindu sages Atreya, Bharadvaja, Kashyapa, Sushruta, Parashara, and Charaka. Sage Atreya's disciple Agnivesha is said to have written the original *Agnivesha Samhita* around 1000 BC which has come down to us in the form of *Charaka Samhita*. This text is considered an authoritative pronouncement of Ayurvedic doctrine. Its present form goes back to the seventh century BC. Sage Charaka defines Ayurveda as 'the science through which one can obtain knowledge about the useful and harmful types of life (*hita* and *ahita ayus*), happy and miserable types of life, things which are useful and harmful for such types of life, the span of life as well as the very nature of life'. Ayurveda thus emphasizes on not only leading a happy life from an individualistic point of view but also aims to be beneficial to society as a whole.

Health, according to Ayurveda, is not merely freedom from disease. It is essential that body, mind and soul are in an excellent state so that the individual can perform his functions and fulfil his role in life which in Vedic philosophy is called *dharma*; and ultimately work towards the final goal of salvation or *moksha* with the help of wealth, economic means which is *artha* and by satisfying his legitimate desires of love and sex which is *kama*. The roots of Indian culture can be traced back to the Vedic period, from c. 5000 BC or perhaps even earlier. All the four Vedas—*Rig, Yajur, Sama, Atharva*—contain several references to the digestive system, metabolism, anatomy and descriptions of diseases along with the bacteria that cause them and most importantly, the concept of *tridosha* or the three doshas. The doshas, according to the Vedas, are subtle elements in the human body responsible for all its functions. According to the dictates of Ayurveda, illnesses occur due to an imbalance in the equilibrium between the three doshas—*vayu, pitta, kapha*. Roughly translated, *vayu* (also known as *vata*) is wind, *pitta* can be represented by bile and *kapha* by phlegm.

In India, a large section of the vast population depends on the indigenous Ayurvedic tradition which has deep cultural roots because of its easy availability, accessibility and reliability. The carriers of this tradition are the millions of housewives brought up in this culture, the hundreds of birth-attendants, bone-setters, village herbalists, those skilled in eye-care, dental care and in the specialized treatment of mental diseases. Ayurveda is a body of knowledge which is extremely coherent and logical within itself yet not restricted by any fixed dogma. Like life itself, it is universal and dynamic.

The Basic Elements

❶ The science of Ayurveda is a branch of Indian philosophy. Although it is deeply rooted in Indian culture, the universality of Indian thought is widely acknowledged. Hence, the world can respond to Ayurveda as a science of healing based on man's response to his environment.

❷ Its universal approach emphasizes its applicability and relevance to all, irrespective of their geographical, cultural and religious differences. As a science, it is founded on the

9

rational principles of physiology, pathology, pharmacology and diagnostics, which have been critiqued, systematized and generalized, based on the rigid principles of logic.

❸ Being a holistic science of life, it believes that the functioning of the body is closely related to the mind and soul of the individual. Ideally speaking, the body should be free from disease, the mind should be happy and the person should be spiritually elevated. It follows, therefore, that certain regimens regarding diet must be observed as also codes of conduct in order to achieve a harmonious life. In prescribing medicines or therapies, Ayurveda takes cognizance of the mind as well as the body.

❹ In Ayurveda, germs and organisms which cause diseases are described as secondary factors. The primary factor is the disturbance in the equilibrium of the three doshas. The doshas: vayu, pitta and kapha are three elementary functional units or principles on which the building up and sustenance of the body depends. They may roughly be represented by the terms, wind for vayu, bile for pitta and phlegm for kapha. But the doshas are not actually these substances. Vayu, pitta, and kapha are more than that. They are forces that cause these substances to be produced in the body. They are the outcome of the absorption of the basic elements in the universe by the human sensory organs.

They exist in all individual constitutions, in certain combinations, endowing each with a characteristic feature. The body generally maintains an equilibrium in the functioning of these doshas. Ayurveda believes that just as seeds sown over barren land will not take root, even virulent germs cannot multiply and produce disease if this equilibrium is maintained in the body. Maintaining good health is as important as treating diseases.

❺ Therapeutic use is made of drugs of vegetable origin, animal products and metals, minerals, gems and semi-precious stones. They are processed only in order to render them non-toxic, palatable and therapeutically more potent. No synthetic additives are used in these processes. The processes themselves have been carefully designed to preserve the therapeutic properties of the medicines' ingredients. Toxic ingredients such as aconite, mercury and arsenic are made to pass through elaborate processes before they are used. Only minute doses are prescribed after their efficacy has been tried and tested over time. Ayurvedic medicines not only cure the patient of diseases, they also provide immunity against future attacks. In normal healthy individuals, they help to revitalize the body cells and stimulate the immune system.

❻ Ayurvedic therapy is directed towards the patient rather than the disease. The line of treatment for two patients suffering from the same disease may differ. The physician prescribes medication and a regimen for each individual patient depending on his/her constitution and mental state. He does not prescribe for the disease alone.

❼ The whole of nature is included in the realm of Ayurveda. The individual is the microcosm of the universe which is the macrocosm. All the elements of the universe can be found in the individual. Hence, the external world is, in a sense, represented in the individual. Because it is based on the elements existing in the universe and the individual's awareness of these, Ayurveda as a science must necessarily comply with the laws of nature. Therefore, Ayurveda and the world around it are inter-dependent. Both the healer and the healed are part of the same ecosystem. Ayurveda is an environment-friendly science which enables the individual to live in harmony with nature and as a part of nature.

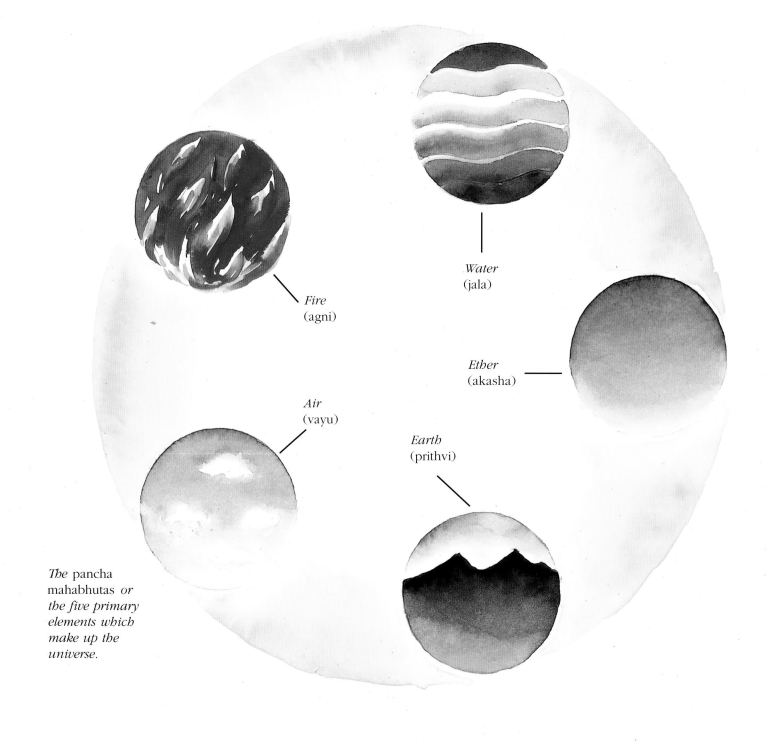

Fire
(agni)

Water
(jala)

Ether
(akasha)

Air
(vayu)

Earth
(prithvi)

The pancha
mahabhutas *or
the five primary
elements which
make up the
universe.*

The Natural Body Constitution

———— ✳ ————

*I*ndian philosophy represents various schools or systems of thought which are known as *darshanas*. Broadly divided, these systems fall into two categories: *astika darshanas* and *nastika darshanas*, the former acknowledge the authority of the Vedas while the latter do not.

The relevance of Ayurveda in today's world lies in the fact that the science is the product of an ancient civilization and culture that postulate man as part of and as the microcosm of the universe, the macrocosm.

The first thing is to realise one's limitations. It should be obvious that the moment once transgresses those limits one falls ill. Thus a balanced diet, eaten in accordance with needs gives one freedom from disease. How is one to know what is the proper diet for one? The purpose of all this is that everyone should be his own doctor and find out his limitations.

. . . Mahatma Gandhi

What this really means is that for Ayurveda, every phenomenon in the universe can be found to take place in the individual, albeit in a subtle form. Every individual act has therefore an impact on the environment (in a very broad sense of the term) and on the universe.

All matter and psyche, from the most subtle to the gross are characterized by three attributes or *gunas*, namely *sattva*, *rajas* and *tamas*. *Sattva* stands for consciousness, *rajas* for energy and dynamism and *tamas* stands for mass, inertia and stability. These three attributes are conceived as real and substantive entities perpetually uniting, separating and reuniting. Everything in the universe is consequent upon their unique arrangement and combination.

In the phenomenal world whatever energy exists is due to *rajas*; all matter, resistance and stability are due to *tamas*, and all manifestations of the consciousness are because of *sattva*. The predominant attribute in a substance becomes manifest while the other two become latent though their presence is felt by their effects. These collocations make for the difference in the psychological temperament and physical constitution of an individual.

An understanding of these three attributes and what they represent is important for appreciating various Ayurvedic concepts. The individual according to the Vedas is made up of five successive layers or *koshas*: the *annamaya kosha* or the physical body; the *pranamaya kosha*: the astral body or the *elan vitae* or what the individual feels; the *manomaya kosha*: the psyche or what the individual thinks; the *vijnanmaya kosha*: the intellect which can discriminate; the *anandamaya kosha*: the sheath of bliss.

The physical body in its turn is composed of five basic elements or *mahabhutas* which make up the universe. These elements are *prithvi, jala, agni, vayu* and *akasha*. Loosely translated, these five elements are often referred to as earth, water, fire, air and ether respectively. They do not, however, connote the correct and full implications of the

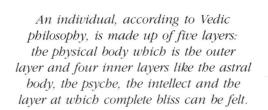

An individual, according to Vedic philosophy, is made up of five layers: the physical body which is the outer layer and four inner layers like the astral body, the psyche, the intellect and the layer at which complete bliss can be felt.

original Sanskrit terms. They are used in a representative sense in order to help understand how the external world is linked to the world within us.

Here it may be useful to elaborate on the five element or *pancha mahabhuta* theory.

Man perceives the external world in five different ways through his five senses (*indriyas*): the auditory, tactile, taste, visual and the olfactory. Through the corresponding sense organs, man not only perceives the external object but also absorbs it into his body in the form of energy.

Each element is composed of all the five elements but each also has one predominant characteristic which gives it its name. For example, ordinary water does not contain water alone. Its composition includes water, air, earth, fire and ether. The force of cohesion or the power of attraction which is inherent in water is its characteristic feature.

Just as the individual body is composed of five elements, so also are food and drugs (and other objects in the world). In the human body, these elements are explained in terms of doshas, tissues or *dhatus* and waste products or *malas*. The meaning and relevance of these words will be explained in detail.

Elements of the Body

The doshas have certain qualities or attributes which characterize their effects on the human body. The individual remains healthy as long as these elements are in a state of equilibrium in the body. The body has the capacity to overcome minor disturbances in their equilibrium. But if this equilibrium is disturbed beyond a point, the body succumbs to disease and decay. The doshas exist in two forms in the body, namely, gross and subtle. In their subtle state, they are beyond the normal cognition of the senses.

Their normal and abnormal states are ascertained by the manifestation of their respective actions. These three doshas control all the physical and psychological functions of an individual. Each one of these doshas is further subdivided into five categories on the basis of their actions on different parts of the body. The details of the actions of the three doshas can be found in Ayurvedic texts. They are briefly stated here.

Vayu or vata is unctuous, light, cold, mobile, abundant in quantity. It is the originator of all movement in the body and it governs, in general, all nervous functions. There are in all eighty kinds of possible disturbances that can occur due to vayu imbalance. Some of these are pain, stiffness,

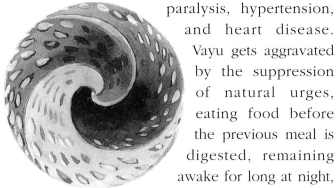

Vayu or wind, one of three vital elements of the body.

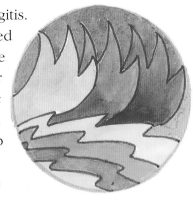

Pitta or bile, one of three vital elements of the body.

paralysis, hypertension, and heart disease. Vayu gets aggravated by the suppression of natural urges, eating food before the previous meal is digested, remaining awake for long at night, excessive shouting, too much physical exercise, excessive jerks when travelling in a vehicle for a long time, intake of ingredients having pungent, bitter and astringent tastes, eating dry food, worry, sexual indulgence, fear, fasting, cold and grief. It also gets aggravated during the onset of the rainy season.

Pitta is a hot, sour and pungent liquid. It mainly governs the enzymes and hormones. Pitta is also responsible for digestion, pigmentation, body temperature, hunger, thirst, sight, courage and so forth. There are forty kinds of possible disturbances caused by pitta imbalance such as a burning sensation, excessive body temperature, blue moles, jaundice, urticaria and pharyngitis. Pitta gets aggravated by excessive intake of pungent and sour things, alcoholic beverages, saline, hot and sharp substances. Other responsible factors are anger, excessive exposure to sun and fire, fear, fatigue, intake of dry vegetables and alkalies. Indigestion and irregular eating habits also aggravate pitta. During autumn, pitta tends to get aggravated.

Kapha is unctuous, smooth, soft, sweet, firm, dense, cold, viscous and clear. Kapha is responsible for the connection and movement of the joints, the solid nature of the body and its sustenance, sexual power, strength, patience and so on. Among the twenty possible disturbances that can be caused by kapha imbalance are anorexia nervosa, laziness, mucous expectoration, hardening of blood vessels, obesity, suppression of digestive power and so forth. Thus the

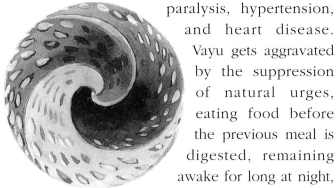

Kapha or phlegm, one of three vital elements of the body.

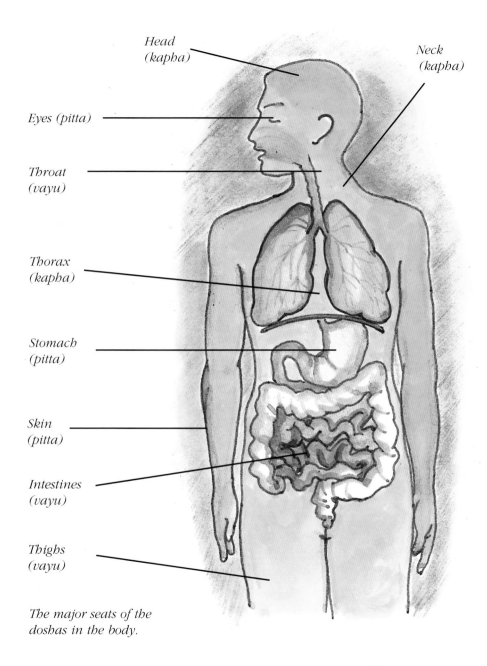

Head (kapha)

Neck (kapha)

Eyes (pitta)

Throat (vayu)

Thorax (kapha)

Stomach (pitta)

Skin (pitta)

Intestines (vayu)

Thighs (vayu)

The major seats of the doshas in the body.

three doshas govern the physico-chemical and physiological activities of the body. Kapha becomes aggravated by sleeping during the day, overeating, by the intake of sweet, cold, heavy and sour things, fish, meat, preparations of sesame, sugarcane and milk, by intake of food and drinks containing excess salt and water and during the spring season.

Doshas are aggravated under certain conditions and diminished under some. Both states lead to disease. They can also be in a state of equilibrium which is a condition of perfect health and is called *sama*.

The three doshas pervade all over the body. There are however some elements or organs of the body in which they are primarily located. For example, the heart, the throat, the urinary bladder, the intestines, the pelvic region, the thighs, the two legs and the bones are the primary seats of vayu. The seats of pitta are the eyes, the skin (perspiration), the lymph, the blood and the stomach. Similarly, the seats of kapha are the thorax, the head, the neck, the joints, the upper portion of the stomach and the fat tissues of August, i.e. at the end of the summer. Pitta gets aggravated between October to December, i.e. during autumn, and kapha gets aggravated between February and April, i.e. during spring. In other countries, while the months of the seasons may vary, the doshas are aggravated by seasonal

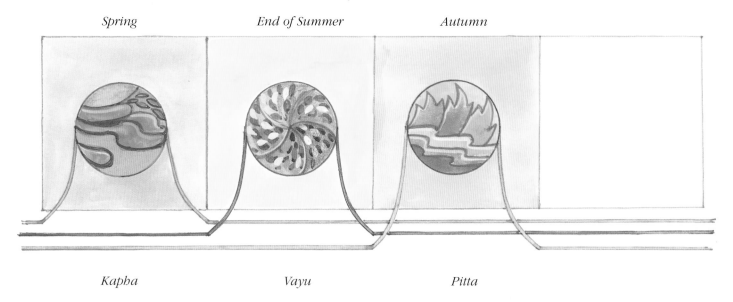

Spring   *End of Summer*   *Autumn*

Kapha   *Vayu*   *Pitta*

This graph shows the relationship between the doshas and the seasons. Vayu-related diseases may occur in the end of summer as that is when vayu is aggravated in the body, pitta is aggravated in autumn and kapha in spring.

the body.

During different seasons of the year, these doshas undergo certain changes. In India, for example, vayu gets aggravated between June and changes. If certain precautionary measures are not taken during these seasons, a person becomes prone to diseases caused by these doshas. These measures include undertaking therapies such as

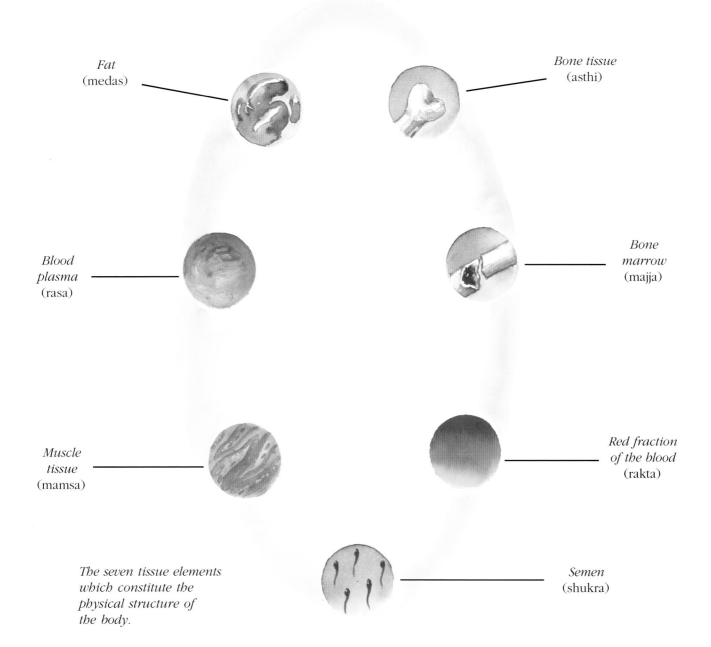

Fat
(medas)

Bone tissue
(asthi)

*Blood
plasma*
(rasa)

*Bone
marrow*
(majja)

*Muscle
tissue*
(mamsa)

*Red fraction
of the blood*
(rakta)

*The seven tissue elements
which constitute the
physical structure of
the body.*

Semen
(shukra)

vomiting, purgation and enema before the onset of certain seasons, following specific regimens during them and taking different herbal preparations to counter the diseases caused by aggravation of the doshas. For example, the herb, *haritaki* (*Terminalia chebula*), may be taken in summer with jaggery, during the rains with rock salt, in autumn with sugar, in early winter with ginger powder, in late winter with the powder of long pepper (*Piper longum*) and in spring with honey.

✽ Tissue Elements

The physical structure of the body is composed of seven categories of tissue elements or *dhatus*, namely, chyle including plasma (*rasa*), red fraction of the blood (*rakta*), muscle tissue (*mamsa*), fat (*medas*), bone tissue (*asthi*), bone marrow (*majja*) and semen or generative fluid (*shukra*). These seven are again composed of the five elements.

Each tissue has its own function in the body and helps to determine the identity of the self within the body. Their functions take place in seven stages, with each paving the way for the succeeding one's function. Thus, soon after the food is ingested into the blood stream, the process of conversion and assimilation begins. The haemoglobin fraction of the blood helps in this process. This then gives way to the nourishment of the flesh or muscle tissue. The fat tissue comes next. This signifies unctuousness and provides warmth and heat. An overabundance of fat can become a disease of the mind and body, just as its opposite can lead to anorexia nervosa. Bone tissue which follows, provides support for the fat in the body. Unlike the four earlier tissue elements, bone is part of the external integrity of the body. Healthy bone tissue and its filling, bone marrow, go together. Bone marrow prevents the hollow bone from being filled with vata. The state of the bone marrow is reflected in the eyes giving them a clear, strong and bright, shining look. The final stage in this series of reactions is the function of semen which is an important element in procreation.

The metabolic transformation of the tissue elements produces a substance called *ojas*. *Ojas* provides immunity or the power to resist attacks of diseases. If *ojas* is destroyed, the body succumbs to death.

✽ Waste Products

Each tissue element is also linked to one or more waste products which are known as *malas*, such as stool, perspiration, ear wax, fatty secretions of the skin, mucous, saliva, discharge from the eyes, and so on. An excess or deficiency in the production of the waste products is indicative of improper or inefficient functioning of the tissue elments and would therefore provoke a disease. The doshas will also then be in a disturbed state with one or more of them aggravated. The regular elimination of waste from the body is essential for maintaining good health.

❧ Enzymes

The role of enzymes or *agnis* which help in the process of digestion and metabolism is all important. Any diminution in their quantity obstructs the channels of circulation in the body and causes disease. There are thirteen enzymes in all in the human body, according to Ayurvedic theory. Their function is to help in the conversion of the food that is ingested into various tissues and thus facilitate assimilation. The power of the enzymes is mild in infancy and increases with age and starts to decline after the age of fifty.

❧ Channels of Circulation

There are innumerable channels of circulation or *srotas* in the body. They carry external nutrient material into the organs and tissues of the body, promote their growth and eliminate metabolic waste. Any obstruction to these channels will give rise to diseases. The three doshas circulate throughout the entire body. The psyche or the mind circulates throughout the conscious parts of the body excluding nails, hair, stool and urine. Any impediment or obstruction in these channels therefore disturbs the equilibrium of the doshas. On the other hand, aggravated doshas can also cause obstruction to these channels. Therefore, the knowledge of these channels is important for the individual's well-being. In Ayurvedic therapeutics, measures are first taken to remove any obstruction to these channels.

Physical Constitution

Ayurveda classifies individuals broadly into seven categories, according to their constitution or *prakriti*, which has specific physical and mental characteristics. These seven categories are an outcome of the dominance of a particular dosha; vayu, pitta and kapha, or of combinations of the three doshas. These basic traits of an individual are developed at the very time of birth and remain until death.

A knowledge of constitution is essential for selecting appropriate food, beverages and other regimens as also for choosing medicines for the treatment of ailments. Furthermore, a person may be more prone to certain kinds of ailments because of his natural constitution or combination of doshas.

Primarily, human constitution is of seven types: ❶ Vata constitution. ❷ Pitta constitution. ❸ Kapha constitution. ❹ Vata-pitta constitution. ❺ Pitta-kapha constitution. ❻ Vata-kapha constitution. ❼ Sama constitution.

The vata, pitta and kapha constitutions refer to constitutions having a dominance of the characteristic features associated with that particular dosha. The mixed constitutions, namely, vata-pitta constitution, pitta-kapha constitution and vata-kapha constitution have the characteristic features of their respective doshas in a combined form. In sama constitution, which is the best, everything is in a state of complete balance.

The characteristic features of a person having vata constitution are: • Dryness and roughness of the skin and the body. • Emaciated body. • Short stature. • Prominence of tendons and veins, roughness of hair, nails, teeth, soles of the feet and palms. • Appearance of cracks in limbs. • Less hair and beard. • Hair with split ends and of brown colour. • Dryness and drowsiness of the eyes.

Some of the characteristic features of an individual with pitta constitution are: • White colour of the skin. • Dryness and tenderness of the body. • Excessive appearance of black moles. • Intense feeling of heat in face and limbs. • Early appearance of grey hair and wrinkles. • Baldness. • Less hair with a reddish brown tinge. • Sloth in muscle movements. • Looseness of the joints. • Body odour. • Coppery colour of nails, eyes, tongue, palate, limbs, palms and soles of the feet. • Enthusiasm. • Small, reddish eyes. • Sparse eyelashes.

Characteristic features of a person having kapha constitution are: • Soft, smooth and unctuous skin. • Compact and muscular body. • White and tender body. • Corpulence. • Compact joints. • White eyes with red tinge at the outer corner. • Curly and black hair. • Prominent forehead, chest and arms. • Beautiful big eyes. • Plenty of eyelashes.

For Ayurvedic treatment, knowledge of individual constitution is very important. For example, a person with a vata constitution will be prone to vata ailments like bronchitis, asthma, common cold, hoarseness of voice, or various diseases of the eye, ear, nose and throat respectively. He or she may have problems of indigestion and diarrhoea and diseases like diabetes. Diseases of other types will not give much trouble to such people.

To prevent the occurrence of diseases, the individual having a vata constitution should always avoid factors which would aggravate vata. He or she should take to vata-alleviating food, drinks and ways of life. Food ingredients which are unctuous and hot are likely to suit such people the most whereas for a person having pitta constitution, cooling things will be most suitable.

Similarly, while administering medicines, a pitta constitution patient is to be given medicines which are cooling and a kapha constitution patient is to be given medicines which bring about a heating effect. Pitta ailments include indigestion, anaemia, and jaundice, besides impairment of vision, skin diseases and psychological disturbances. Kapha ailments include impairment of digestion and of taste. There may be loss of memory and impairment of the functions of sense organs as also a tendency to have pain and malfunctioning in the joints.

Individuals with constitutions dominated by a mixture of two doshas are characterised by the combination of the manifestations of representative doshas. A sama type of individual has all the doshas in a state of equilibrium and is endowed with the good qualities of all the types of individuals described above. Thus, persons having different types of constitutions are vulnerable to some specific diseases, which can be healed by a particular kind of therapy.

Health, according to Ayurveda, is not merely freedom from disease but a state of being in which the individual enjoys physical, mental and spiritual happiness and fulfillment over a relatively uninterrupted period of time. This state of being can only be experienced if all the aspects of the constitution are in a state of balance. The external manifestations of this balance can be explained in terms of the individual's experience of hunger, thirst, sleep and ability to perform his or her normal functions at work and at home without undue strain on the body or mind. The normal human urges such as hunger, thirst and sleep help indicate that the bodily functions of digestion, metabolism and elimination are being performed smoothly.

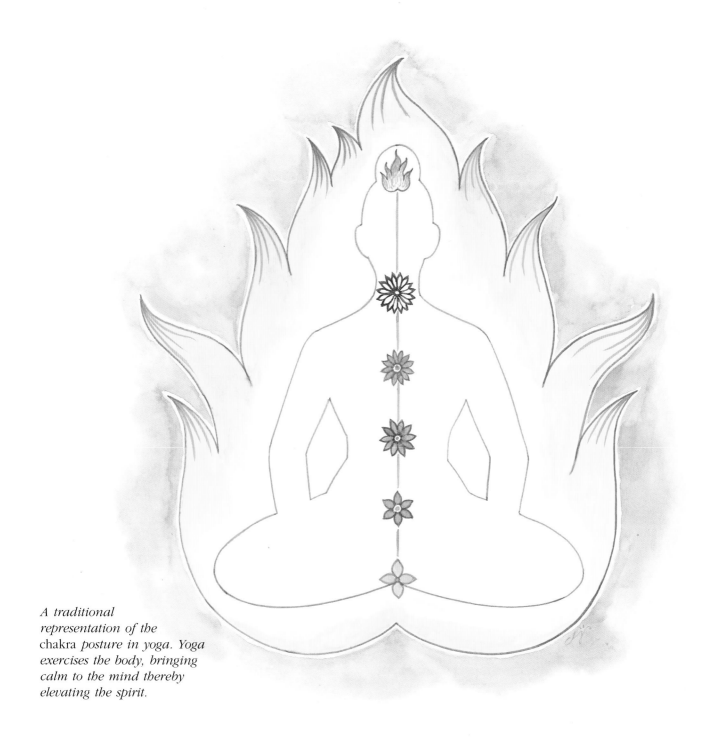

A traditional representation of the chakra *posture in yoga. Yoga exercises the body, bringing calm to the mind thereby elevating the spirit.*

Causes and Diagnosis of Diseases

———— ✳ ————

Understanding our individual constitution, as we have seen, is one of the main ways of keeping good health. Diseases, according to Ayurveda, are caused by an imbalance in the three doshas. The predominance of a dosha in an individual's constitution indicates his or her vulnerability to a particular disease. Diseases in Ayurveda are classified according to the origin of their causes.

Diseases which originate from factors within the human body, including psychosomatic diseases, are called *adhyatmika*. *Adhyatmika* diseases are further

A man who commands his senses and vanquishes his body, who sees one's atman as the atman in all, who purifies his mind before he performs his deeds—such a man is not sullied.

. . . The Bhagvad Gita

divided into hereditary diseases, congenital diseases and those caused by the aggravation of the doshas. *Adhibhautika* diseases are those whose origin can be traced to external physical factors such as germs and accidents. *Adhidaiveka* diseases are caused by the seasons, planetary influences, providential causes and so forth.

The physician diagnoses a disease in an individual by an examination of the patient based on three general methods. These methods are common to understanding any phenomenon in the universe.

25

Direct observation or *pratyaksha*: This is done through the senses: seeing, hearing, smelling, touching and tasting. A direct contact between the senses and the object of examination is thus established.

Inference or *anumana*: Just as one deduces that there is a fire when one sees smoke, one can make deductions from the observation of certain substances under a microscope. For instance, the examination of stool under a microscope will give clues about the state of the health of a person.

Authoritative statement or *shabda*: Experts have bequeathed to us a legacy of authoritative statements regarding diseases. The patient is interrogated closely to determine the exact nature of the disease. The patient's relatives too are questioned for in this way the patient's previous history of diseases can be recorded. Fortified with the knowledge about the disease from previously recorded cases and the findings of experts, the physician can make a diagnosis.

Following these three principles, a brief examination of a patient proceeds in three stages: visual observation or *darshana*, touch or *sparshana*, interrogation or *prashna*. Another important tool of diagnosis in Ayurveda involves the eight-fold method of examination or *ashtasthana pariksha* which has the following steps:

❶ Examination of the pulse or *nadi pariksha*: Pulse examination is carried out with the help of the radial artery. The index, middle and ring fingers of the right hand are used in pulse examination. The index finger is placed about the width of the patient's wrist below the root of the

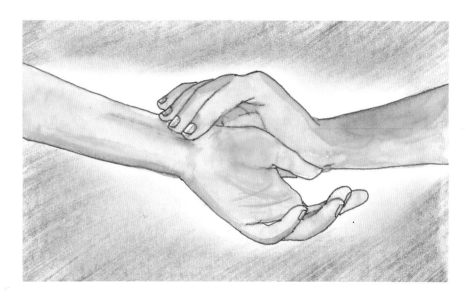

Pulse examination or nadi pariksha *is one of the oldest forms of diagnosis in medicine, whether traditional or modern.*

thumb, the other two fingers are placed next to the index.

Certain rules have to be observed in pulse examination. (a) The examination should be carried out preferably early in the morning after ablutions, on an empty stomach. The pulse should not be examined immediately after a bath or oil massage, nor when the patient is hungry or thirsty. The examination can also be carried out in the afternoon only if the patient has not eaten for three hours. (b) The pulse on the right hand of men and the left hand of women must be examined. (c) The doctor has to have total concentration. (d) The examination of the pulse is repeated at least three times. Each time the pulse is gently and evenly pressed, then the pressure is released. It is important that the doctor feels the pulse of the patient and not the capillaries of his own fingers. (e) The pressure of the examining fingers has to be uniform.

The state of vayu is indicated by the pulse felt with the index finger. The state of pitta is indicated by the pulse felt with the middle finger. The state of kapha is indicated by the pulse felt with the ring finger. The physician should wash his hands each time he has examined a pulse, so that the energies are not transmitted.

If all three doshas are aggravated (the state of *sannipata*), the pulse movement resembles that of a woodpecker. A healthy person's pulse is slow steady and regular. A regular pulse beat of thirty times always indicates good prognosis. While examining the pulse some other factors must also be taken into consideration: vayu content in the body increases in old age, in the late afternoon, late at night, two hours after eating, during summer or in the beginning of the rainy season. Pitta content goes up during youth and middle age, at noon, at midnight, while digesting food and in autumn and the amount of kapha in the body is more in the morning, in the evening, immediately after eating and in spring. Children have more kapha in their bodies. During pregnancy, which is a bi-cardiac stage, there is a kind of a double pulse.

❷ Examination of physical features: Vayu-dominated patients normally have a rather dry and cracked skin and dry hair. They do not like cold things. Pitta-dominated patients are frequently thirsty and hungry. Their skin is hot to touch and often yellowish. The palms and soles are frequently coppery in colour. They have somewhat less hair. Kapha-dominated patients have compact joints, bones and muscles. They are never excessively thirsty or hungry.

❸ Examination of the eyes: In case of vayu diseases, the patient will complain of a burning sensation in the eyes. The eyes will also be dry and smoky. Pitta type of diseases will manifest in a yellowish tinge in the whites of the eyes, an aversion to light and a burning sensation. Unctuous and dull eyes indicate kapha predominance.

❹ Examination of the tongue: Vayu aggravation is indicated when the tongue is cold, rough and cracked. A red or bluish tinge indicates pitta aggravation. And a white and slimy tongue indicates kapha aggravation. The tongue is dark with thorny eruptions when all the doshas are aggravated.

❺ Examination of the skin: A cold skin indicates vayu aggravation. When the skin is hot to touch, pitta is aggravated and a moist and wet skin indicates kapha aggravation.

❻ Examination of nails: Cracked and dry nails indicate vayu aggravation, while red or yellowish nails indicate pitta aggravation.

❼ Urine examination

❽ Stool examination

Applying these methods of examination, an experienced physician is able to comprehend a general impression about the patient's individual constitution and which dosha or combination of doshas is affected. The treatment can thus be broadly identified.

The physician may ask the patient a few questions. For example, if the physician feels that a headache may be caused by a stomach problem he may ask the patient about the food he ate the previous night. Interrogation is thus also a tool of investigation and diagnosis. Ayurvedic classics caution the physician against being very specific in naming the disease in a patient. Names are attributed to some diseases purely in order to facilitate and aid the physician in ascertaining and understanding the entire gamut of the remaining diseases for which names are not furnished.

It is however essential to determine the exact nature of a disease in order to prescribe the proper treatment. Each disease must be studied with regard to the following points:

• Causes of diseases or *nidana*.
• The premonitory signs or symptoms or *purvarupa*.
• The actual signs or symptoms or *rupa*.
• Exploratory therapy or *upasaya*.
• The mode of manifestation of the disease or *samprapti*.

Causes of diseases may vary. Some factors may cause diseases to appear quite early; others may have delayed effects; yet others may not be strong enough to cause disease. There are also some which cause instantaneous effects, for example strong poisons. Various types of diets, regimens and the effects of the seasons are exogenous factors which cause disease. The endogenous ones are attributed to the vitiation of the doshas and tissue elements.

Premonitory signs can be general or specific in indicating the nature of the disease that will manifest itself. They provide a clue to the diagnosis of the impending disease. At this stage some diet restrictions as well as administration of medicines may avert the onset of the actual disease.

Exploratory therapy is carried out to arrive at the correct diagnosis of a disease of doubtful identity. Actual signs and symptoms of the disease become manifest if it is not averted during the premonitory stage. The signs and the symptoms of the disease are related to the site of its origin or *udbhava sthana*, the site of its manifestation or *adhisthana* and the path of transportation or *sanchara marga*. All actual signs and symptoms are also related to the doshas, tissues, enzymes and channels of circulation. The importance of identifying these three aspects for treatment becomes apparent in the examples discussed here.

❧ Asthma

Asthma can be of many types but the most common variety is bronchial asthma known as *tamaka swasa* in Ayurveda. In most cases, either at the beginning of the disease or before each attack, the patient suffers from indigestion, constipation or even diarrhoea. In Ayurveda, asthma is supposed to originate from an affliction of the stomach and other parts of the gastro-intestinal tract. The seat of manifestation is the lungs though the pressure causes the heart to get involved. Nasal congestion, even obstruction and sneezing are experienced before an attack of asthma. In Ayurveda, therefore, both for the prevention and cure of bronchial asthma, primary attention is given to the stomach, bowels, nose and lungs. Simultaneously, in chronic cases, care is taken to strengthen the heart.

❧ Rheumatism

In rheumatism, the site of origin of the disease is the colon while the site of manifestation lies in the joints. Rheumatism is a disease marked by inflammation and pain in the joints and muscles, usually recurrent and often caused by exposure to cold. It is also at times associated with fever. If the disease is not identified and treated in time, it can affect the heart. Known as *amavata* in Ayurveda, the disease is caused by the production and circulation of a substance called *ama* in the body. *Ama* is introduced in the body as a result of improper digestion and metabolism. It accumulates in the joints and causes inflammation and pain. In general, patients with a tendency towards constipation and those who are prone to irregular diets are affected by *amavata*.

❧ Influenza

Influenza is an infectious disease marked by depression, fever, acute catarrhal inflammation of the nose, the larynx and the bronchi, neuralgic and muscular pains, gastro-intestinal disorders and nervous disturbances. This disease is caused by a virus and often occurs in epidemic form during seasonal changes. It is known as *vata slaishmika jwara*. During seasonal changes, particularly with the coming of the rains, the equilibrium of doshas in a normal individual gets slightly disturbed. Persons who are prone to constipation and a morbidity of the nasal mucous membranes or throat are more likely than others to fall prey to this disease.

❧ Headache

Ayurveda considers headaches to be of various kinds depending on the predominance of the dosha involved in the pathogenesis of this disease. The causative factors can be both physical and pyschological. Defective eye-sight, inflammation of the sinus, high blood pressure, sleeplessness, brain tumour, prolonged overwork, emotional strain, exposure to excessive heat, indigestion, constipation and several other factors can cause headache. Headache is a symptom of many other diseases like fever, influenza and bronchitis.

The signs and symptoms associated with headache vary with the aggravation of each dosha. Thus there are headaches associated with a heavy head, running nose, watery eyes and so on, those which happen particularly in the early hours of the morning, during the rainy season or in the winter, and immediately after a meal. In summer and autumn, headaches are often associated with a burning sensation in the head and bleeding from the nose. This is the pitta type of headache. The vata type of headache is always associated with giddiness, dryness and roughness of the eyes and pain in different parts of the head.

❧ Migraine

Another type of headache which is characterized by paroxysmal attacks and occurs in bouts is migraine. The patient often feels intense pain only on one side of the head and manages to lead a perfectly normal life between attacks. The primary cause of such headaches is generally considered to be excessive worry and anxiety. Exposure to the heat of the sun, cold winds or snow for a considerable length of time precipitates this headache. Patients of migraine also suffer from sinusitis. Heaviness of the head and nasal congestion in a mild form are experienced between attacks. Nausea accompanies this intense pain in the head and vomiting eases the pain. Patients suffering from migraine are usually constipated, and have to be treated for this. Both body and mind are involved in this disease which is primarily psychosomatic. In the following chapter, some common diseases are analysed and their treatment outlined.

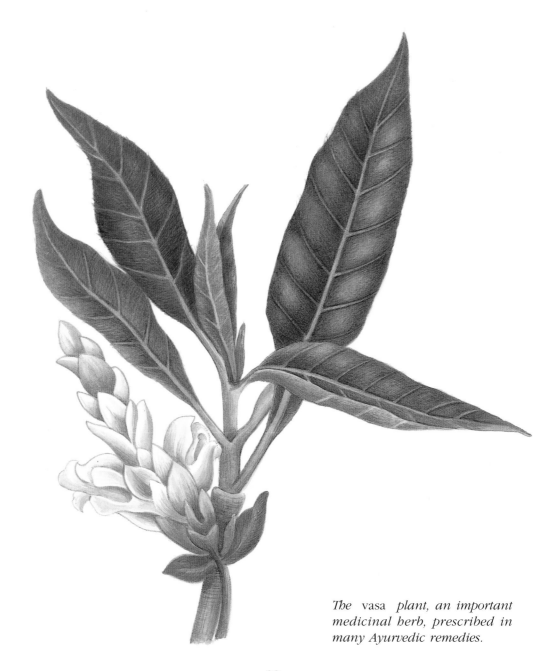

The vasa *plant, an important medicinal herb, prescribed in many Ayurvedic remedies.*

Treatment of Disease

———— * ————

*A*yurveda looks upon food and drugs as having similar effects on the human body. Food and drugs are composed of the same five elements that are found in nature. Therefore, the components of both can be categorized according to these five elements. Thus, even if these drugs are continued after the body has regained its normal state, they can provide immunity against disease by strengthening the system in much the same way as a tonic does.

Symptomatic treatment is almost alien to Ayurvedic medicine. The disease as a whole, including the site of its origin and the site of its manifestation, is

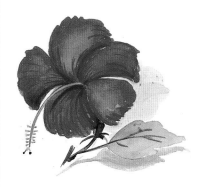

Some offer the work of the body and the vital breath of life, in the fire of self control, lit by knowledge.

. . . The Bhagvad Gita

taken into consideration for the choice of treatment. The primary aim of treatment is to break the process of pathogenesis. It is only when the symptoms become excessively painful that the Ayurvedic physician resorts to symptomatic treatment.

Chronic diseases, ailments of the mind and the body will naturally involve a lengthy process of therapy accompanied by a fairly strict adherence to diet and regimen. Recovery will necessarily be a slow and gradual process. Usually, the patient opts for Ayurvedic treatment after other systems have been tried and failed.

As we have already

emphasized, even before a diagnosis is formed and the treatment of a patient is begun, it is essential to identify the patient's individual constitution.

In general, three types of therapies are used in Ayurveda to correct a dosha imbalance. These constitute internal cleansing, external cleansing and surgical therapy. Where diseases of the mind are discerned, psychotherapy is employed. Medicines meant for internal cleansing, as a rule, are used to treat diseases caused by improper diet which can include excessively rich food, food eaten at irregular hours, stale food and so on. External cleansing which has a curative effect includes massage, fomentation and unction and entails external contact with the body. Surgical therapy comprises excision, incision, puncturing, scraping, uprooting, rubbing with a rough surfaced substance, suturing, probing and application of leeches and alkalies.

Ayurveda believes that propitiating the Supreme Power which controls the universe and warding off evil spirits will give the mind peace and sanity. Hence, Ayurvedic psychotherapy is administered through *homa* or the act of offering oblations like pouring clarified liquid butter or *ghee* into a sacred fire, fasting, the performance of propitiatory and religious rites, offering prayers to the gods and to Hindu priests or *brahmans* who chant prayers for the patient's welfare.

The Ayurvedic physician, in prescribing a therapy, examines both the patient and the disease carefully. The selection of medicines depends upon several factors:

Doshas: These may get diminished or aggravated in quantity. Seasonal changes, the constitution of the individual and the tissue elements affected by the disease also influence variation in the doshas.

The nature of the drugs: The drug prescribed may vary in its effect due to the age, feature and the combination of constituent herbs. Drugs also vary in their effectiveness by virtue of their qualities: taste, potency, post-digestive effect and the specific action the drug provokes.

Time: Treatment may vary according to changes in seasons, the time of day and night, or duration of the disease.

Strength: The patient's strength or general resistance to disease is a factor which influences the selection of the treatment.

Body Structure: The patient's body may be fat, lean, porous or loose-limbed or compact. The condition of the vital organs may differ too.

Diet: The kind of food the patient eats may affect the selection of the drug. The way the food is prepared, the quantity which the patient eats are important factors in choosing a drug.

Mental State: The patient's mind may be affected with grief, fear or happiness. This would influence the choice of medicine.

Age: Different stages of life such as infancy, youth, old age may also cause variations in the treatment selected.

Depending on the kind of disease, Ayurveda offers therapies, which are of six types:

- Lightening therapy or *Langhana.*
- Nourishing therapy or *Brimhana.*
- Oleation therapy or *Snehana.*
- Fomentation therapy or *Svedana.*
- Drying therapy or *Rukshana.*
- Astringent therapy or *Stambhana.*

Lightening therapy can include the administration of six types of elimination therapies such as emesis, purgation, enema and inhalation; control of thirst; exposure to wind and sun; intake of drugs that stimulate digestion; fasting; and physical exercise. These are specialized therapies where herbal decoctions and medicated oils are utilized. Elimination therapies can be judiciously used in the case of patients who tend to be corpulent and who suffer from diseases which are caused by aggravated kapha, pitta, and vata and affect the blood and excreta.

Drugs that promote digestion are useful in treating diseases such as vomiting, nausea and anorexia, diarrhoea, heart diseases, cholera, intestinal disorders, fever, constipation, belching, heaviness of the body caused by a vitiation of kapha and pitta. Fasting and control of thirst will take care of the same diseases in less effective ways. Such diseases which are mild or moderate in strong individuals can be cured by physical exercise and exposure to a conducive climate. Lightening therapy can be administered during winter (November to February) to patients suffering from skin diseases, obstinate urinary disorders, and those who possess a corpulent body together with unctuousness and fluidity. It can also be prescribed for those who suffer from diseases of vitiated vata.

Nourishing therapy can be used effectively for those suffering from emaciation, phthisis, weakness, old age, exertion from long tours and habitual indulgence in sex and alcohol. Such persons are in greater need of this therapy during summer. The kind of nourishing food prescribed for this therapy consists of fresh meat of young animals, fish and birds which have been nurtured on natural feed and slaughtered accordingly. Patients afflicted with piles, sprue or consumption are recommended soups of meat-eating birds and animals, rendered light for easy digestion. Unction, sleep, enema with sweet-tasting drugs, sugar, milk and *ghee* constitute universal nourishing devices.

Oleation therapy uses *ghee*, oil, muscle fat and bone marrow. This therapy is usually done in three ways: oral administration, administration through the anus with a syringe and massage. The

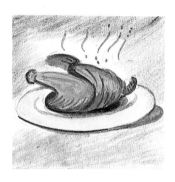

Nourishing therapy provides strength to patients of emaciation and phthisis.

simplest way is to drink hot sweetened milk with one or two teaspoonfuls of *ghee* before going to bed. *Ghee* is the best because of its power to effectively assimilate the properties of drugs boiled in it. *Ghee* alleviates pitta and vata and is conducive to blood and semen. It has a cooling effect on the body. It also has a softening effect and adds to the clarity of the voice and the complexion. Oil alleviates vata but does not aggravate kapha. It promotes bodily strength and is beneficial for the skin. It is a hot substance, also a stabiliser and it controls the morbidity of the female genital organs. Muscle fat is prescribed for the treatment of injury, fracture, trauma, prolapse of the uterus, earache and headache. It enhances the virility of a person. It is also useful for those who do physical exercise. Bone marrow enhances strength, semen, kapha,

fat and the marrow. It adds to the physical strength of the individual, especially of the bones.

Ghee should be taken in autumn, muscle fat and bone marrow in the months of April and May and oil during the rainy season. One should not take any of the unctuous substances when it is either extremely hot or cold.

Fomentation therapy is of thirteen kinds in Ayurveda. This therapy induces perspiration thereby eliminating toxins from the skin. The simplest way to perspire is to wrap oneself in a towel after a hot bath and lie covered till the body stops perspiring. Other methods are to apply external heat like a hot water bottle, hot sand bags and heated stones. Fomentation is used to cure coryza, cough, hiccups, dyspnoea, heaviness of the body, pain in the ears, neck and head, hoarseness of voice, spasmodic obstruction in the throat, paralysis of the face,

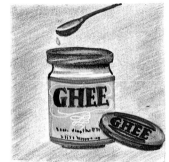

Drinking hot milk with ghee is important in oleation therapy.

limbs, the whole body or part of it. It can also help when there is distension of the abdomen;

constipation and suppression of urine; stiffness of sides, back, waist and abdomen; sciatica; dysuria; enlargement of the scrotum; pain and stiffness of feet, knee, calf; oedema; neuralgia of the upper and lower extremities; diseases due to impaired digestion and metabolism.

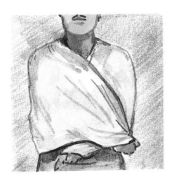

Perspiration induced by fomentation removes toxins from the body.

Drying therapy involves the intake of pungent, bitter and astringent substances like cakes made of mustard and sesame, as also honey. Sexual indulgence is prescribed. This therapy is recommended for patients suffering from diseases where the channels of circulation are obstructed and there is an excessive dominance of the aggravated dosha which is manifested in the vital organs of the body through spasticity of the thighs, gout and severe urinary disorders.

Astringent therapy is a therapy which reduces or prevents excessive physiological secretions. It can be applied in case of uncontrolled watering of eyes, excessive secretion of ear-wax, profuse menstrual flow and diarrhoea. Ayurveda considers substances like spinach and dates astringent which decrease pitta and kapha but increase vata.

The drugs used in the treatment of diseases whether they are oils, powders or liquids, work along the lines indicated in the six types of therapies that have been outlined in this chapter. A detailed description of some of the herbs and other substances used in the treatment of a few select diseases follows.

The Ayurvedic physician precribes certain **standard therapies** keeping in mind the factors discussed above for diseases whose drugs are common and easily available in Ayurvedic centres. However, in every culture there are innumerable little tips and recipes for health care that have survived the test of time and become a part of family folk-lore. Where indigenous systems of medicine are still followed, such instances are numerous and a part of the lives of the people inhabiting those regions. In Ayurveda, therefore there are also a few **home remedies** that can be safely tried out.

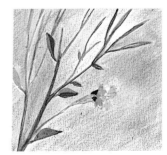

Drying therapy prescribes pungent and astringent foods comprising mustard.

Standard Therapies

❧ Bronchial Asthma

Bronchial asthma or *tamaka swasa*, the most common respiratory disease is considered to originate from an affliction of the stomach and other parts of the gastro-intestinal tract, though it

Haritaki *and* amalaki, *perhaps the most important Ayurvedic plants, the fruits of which are very effective in curing bronchial asthma.*

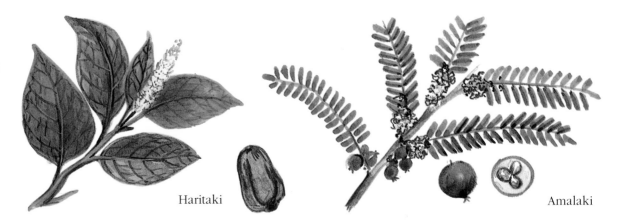

Haritaki

Amalaki

rasayana, both Ayurvedic recipes used as tonics, are commonly used in treatment. The chief ingredient of Chyavanaprasha is the fruit of *amalaki (Emblica officinalis)*, a medicinal plant. This is an important source of Vitamin C. Unlike citrus fruits, the Vitamin C content in *amalaki* does not get destroyed even after boiling for a considerable period. The fruit of *haritaki (Terminalia chebula)* is the main ingredient

manifests itself in the lungs. In most of the cases, therefore, either in the beginning of the disease or before each attack, the patient suffers from indigestion, constipation or even diarrhoea. It is important then to attend to the stomach, bowels, nose and lungs. In chronic cases, care should be taken to strengthen the heart.

Treatment: Chyavanaprasha and Agastya

of the other medicine, Agastya rasayana. Chyavanaprasha is used more as a tonic and is specifically prescribed for bronchial asthma patients who are emaciated and weak. Those who are constipated and also those who often complain of sneezing, blocking of the nostrils and congestion of the throat, are given Agastya rasayana. It usually takes two to three weeks for them to act fully. In chronic cases, they may take still more time. However, they reduce the acuteness of the attack immediately making the duration of the attack comparatively shorter. Even the gap between two attacks will increase and the patient will have time to restore his health in order to successfully fight the next attack.

Other medicines contain mineral products and are useful in reducing the attacks of asthma immediately. They are Shvasa kasa chintamani rasa, Suvarna pushpasuga rasa, Kanakasava, all Ayurvedic recipes made of various medicinal herbs and readily available in Ayurvedic clinics and centres. These medicines may, at times, produce side-effects. Therefore, they should preferably be taken under the supervision of an expert physician.

Diet and regimen: Yogurt, butter-milk, bananas, guavas and fried food should be strictly avoided. A light supper is advised. Avoid smoking, hard exercise, and reduce the intake of tea or coffee to not more than two cups a day. Alcoholic beverages are permitted but in small quantities. Protection is necessary from rain and severe cold winds.

☙ Bronchitis

Bronchitis or *kasa roga* is caused primarily by the impairment of digestion. For the treatment of bronchitis, therefore, physicians choose drugs having properties to correct the functions of both the lungs and the stomach.

Treatment: Whatever the cause may be, the simplest treatment is a teaspoonful of turmeric powder mixed with a cup of warm milk, two to three times a day, depending upon the severity of the condition. It is more effective if taken on an empty stomach. This is an absolutely harmless recipe which can be given to any patient irrespective of age, sex or condition of the disease. Another popular recipe, commonly used as a household remedy for this condition is dried ginger, long pepper and black pepper which are powdered and mixed in equal quantities. Half a teaspoonful of this mixture can be taken three to four times a day, depending upon the severity of the disease. The powder can also be added to tea or coffee. The juice of *vasa* (*Adhatoda vasica*), a medicinal plant, is very useful in curing cough and bronchitis, specially when they become chronic.

All these medicines, taken together promote digestion and metabolism in the body. Simultaneously, they help in the expectoration of the accumulated phlegm and make breathing easy. They also cure fever which accompanies infection because of their anti-pyretic and stimulant effects.

Diet and regimen: Yoghurt and fruits like guavas and bananas should be avoided.

❧ Heart Disease

The functions of the heart and mind are linked in Ayurveda. Irregular and intemperate behaviour patterns and food habits are responsible for many of our present-day heart ailments. Known as

Long pepper (left), ginger (middle) and black pepper (right) taken together is an ancient remedy for bronchitis.

hridroga, heart diseases are classified into several types depending upon the characteristic features of the pain. If the pain is acute, and of a shifting nature, it is called *vatika hridroga* as it is connected to vata vitiation. If it is associated with a burning sensation, then it is a pitta or *paittika hridroga*. In *kaphaja hridroga* or heart disease of kapha type, the pain is usually very mild and is associated with heaviness, nausea and cough. If the heart ailments are caused by invading organisms, they are called *krimija*. They are associated with extreme debility, prostration, giddiness and emaciation.

Treatment: Eleven medical plants are generally used for treatment of heart ailments. A few are described here. They promote the health of the heart and prevent heart diseases, as also cure the manifested signs and symptoms of the various types of heart diseases.

Wood apple or *bael* fruit (*Aegle marmelos*) can act as a heart tonic and cure heart ailments. It is one of the ingredients of Dasamula-satpalaka ghee, an Ayurvedic recipe used for *vatika* and *kaphaja* heart ailments, and Garlic is useful in different types of heart ailments including weakness of heart muscles, in reducing levels of cholesterol, and in preventing blood clotting. *Amalaki* too is used in the treatment of heart ailments, especially those related to irregular blood pressure. Regular intake of this fruit makes the heart healthy and strengthens its muscles.

The leaves of basil (*Ocimum sanctum*), and basil juice strengthen the heart and nerves. The bark of *Arjuna (Terminalia arjuna)*, useful in angina, stimulates the heart, increases blood circulation, nourishes the heart muscles, regulates the heart beat and prevents clotting in the coronary arteries. Its powder is given to the patient during and even after the attack. Arjunarishta, another Ayurvedic tonic, commonly used by physicians, is a derivative of *arjuna*.

Diet and regimen: Fried food, pulses and groundnut oil are prohibited. However, almond and sesame oil are allowed. Cow's milk, *ghee*, and butter are useful for such patients. Stimulants like tea, coffee and alcoholic drinks are very harmful. Both wheat and rice are good for the heart but the former is better. Among pulses, *mung (Phaseolus mungo)* and *masoor (Lens culinaris)* are useful Butter-milk is better than curd or yoghurt. Honey and jaggery should be preferred over purified sugar. Radish, plantain, bitter gourd, pumpkin, cabbage, spinach, lettuce, coriander leaves, onion, carrots, tomato and cucumber are useful too although cauliflower, brinjal and mustard leaves are harmful.

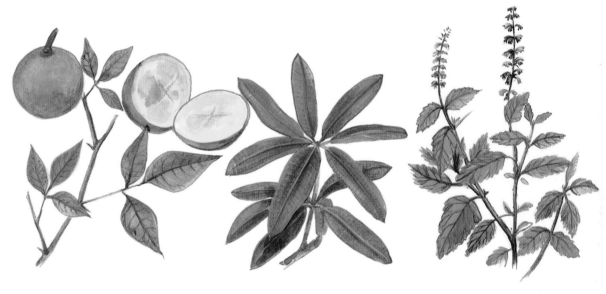

Bael *fruit (left),* arjuna *(middle) and basil (right).* Bael *fruit is an effective heart tonic, basil leaves strengthen the nerves and* arjuna *curbs angina by regulating the heart beat.*

Spices like cumin seeds, black pepper, turmeric, coriander seeds, clove, cardamom, ginger, onion, garlic and asafoetida are very useful but chillies can cause harm. Fruits like banana, papaya, mango, coconut, lychees, black berries, orange, pineapple,

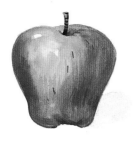

Apple *is considered very good for the heart.*

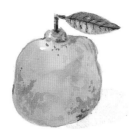

Oranges *are prescribed for patients with a high blood pressure.*

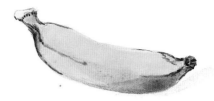

Bananas *are useful for patients suffering from hysteria and heart disease.*

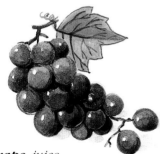

Grape *juice should be taken regularly during jaundice.*

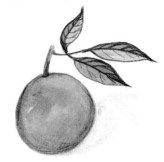

Bael *fruit is one of the best tonics for the heart.*

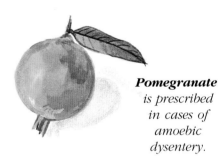

Pomegranate *is prescribed in cases of amoebic dysentery.*

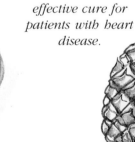

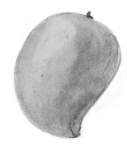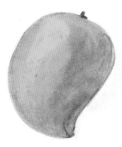

Ripe **papaya** *is one of the best cures for constipation.*

Pineapple *is an effective cure for patients with heart disease.*

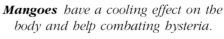

Mangoes *have a cooling effect on the body and help combating hysteria.*

melon, water melon, plums, pomegranate, olives, wood apple, apple, dates, grapes and raisins are useful. But guava, jack fruit and tamarind can harm the heart.

The patient's bowels should be cleaned regularly. A daily walk and a glass of water kept in a copper vessel for twelve hours and taken on an empty stomach early in the morning are beneficial.

☙ High Blood Pressure

Blood pressure varies from person to person depending upon their age, sex, physical and mental work done by them. Older males and those who are exposed to more mental and physical work than normal maintain a higher blood pressure than others. In young people, damage to the functioning of the kidneys may cause high blood pressure. Excessive intake of salt, lack of exercise, mental worry, sleeplessness, among others, are responsible for high blood pressure.

Treatment: All medicines which alleviate vayu and strengthen the nervous system are useful in this condition. Garlic is an excellent drug as it produces a heating effect on the body when taken raw. Garlic made into a paste and mixed with butter-milk is very effective in treating this condition. *Sarpagandha* (*Rauwolfia serpentina*) is a common drug used very widely also in the allopathic system of medicine. In Ayurveda, the whole root of this drug is used in its raw state.

For patients suffering from chronic hypertension, dhara therapy in which various kinds of oil or *taila* are used, is considered to be the most effective. The patient lies on his back and Kshirabala taila, a

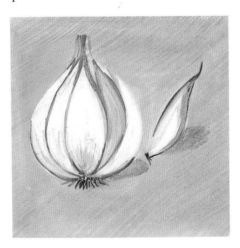

Garlic is the best remedy for patients with high blood pressure.

medicated oil is made to drip on his forehead (between the eye-brows) from a small hole made at the bottom of an earthen vessel. This is done once every day preferably in the morning for about half an hour. This therapy enables the patient to sleep soundly at night and the blood pressure gradually comes down. The same oil is also used for massaging the head as well as the body. A few drops can also be taken internally.

Diet and regimen: Spicy food, hydrogenated oils should be strictly avoided, though butter prepared

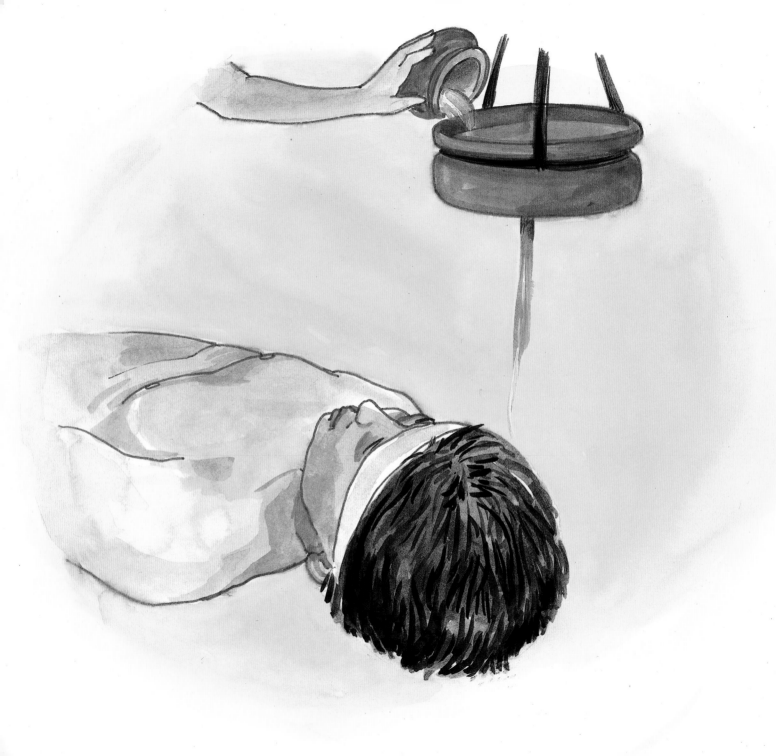

from cow's milk is permitted. Vegetables like bitter gourd and drumsticks which help to clear the bowels are useful. Yellow varieties of pumpkin should be avoided. All types of dry fruits, oranges, bananas, guavas and apples are helpful. Inhaling almond oil or almond oil taken in a cup of warm milk helps in soothing the nerves and thus reduces blood pressure. Fruits and boiled vegetables are considered better than cereals and pulses.

❧ Jaundice

Jaundice or *kamala*, is characterised by the appearance of an yellow tinge in the eyes and skin. It is caused by excessive accumulation of pitta in the blood. The liver is responsible for the production of pitta. If there is any obstruction in the bile duct, or impairment of the functions of the liver, or excessive destruction of the red blood cells, then pitta appears in excess in the blood. Normally it comes out of the body through urine and stool. If, however, there is an obstruction in the bile ducts, then it does not come out through the bowels. Stool gets its characteristic colour because of the bile and if there is an obstruction

Facing page: Dhara therapy makes a hypertense patient lie on his/her back and a medicated oil is made to drip on the forehead through a hole in an earthenware vessel.

in the bile duct then the stool becomes pale-white in colour. The urine becomes excessively yellow in all types of jaundice.

Other manifested symptoms depend upon the cause of the jaundice. The digestion, specially that of fat, is impaired, and consequently the patient becomes physically weak. Destruction of red blood cells and circulation of excessive bile pigments during the oxidation of the tissue cells which results in defective metabolism, occur. The body may experience itching all over.

Treatment: Purgation is carried out in the beginning. Since the patient is generally weak, only mild purgatives like *trivit (Operculina turpethum)*, and *katuki (Picrorhiza kurroa)* which stimulate the function of the liver and increase the flow of bile in the bile duct are used. The root bark of *trivit* and the rhizome of *katuki* are used separately or mixed together in a powder form. Avipattikara churna, a herbal mixture, is also used to cure jaundice. *Bhumyamalaki (Phyllanthus niruri)* is commonly used in the treatment of all types of jaundice. It is a small herb about six inches high with a slender, soft stalk.

Diet and regimen: Plenty of sweet foods and liquids like orange juice and the juice of dry grapes ought to be taken to increase urination and thus elimination of the excessive bile pigments in the blood. Vegetable and meat soups, bitter tasting vegetables like bitter gourds are good. Although sour, pungent and spicy food should be avoided, pomegranate, even if sour, is advised. While curd is harmful, large quantities of fat-free butter-milk are allowed. Alcohol in any form is strictly prohibited. The patient should take complete rest

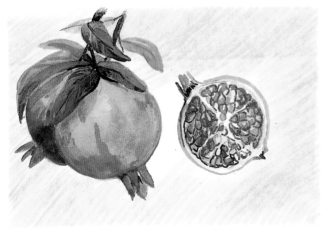

Pomegranate fruit as well as fruit juice is advised for patients suffering from jaundice.

and avoid excessive exposure to the sun as well as sex, anger and anxiety.

ᕙ Oedema

Oedema or non-inflammatory swelling takes place due to several reasons. Ailments of the heart, liver and kidney, as well as anaemia, are some of the important causes of oedema. In all types of oedema, whatever the cause, excess water accumulates inside the tissues. This has to be taken out of the body.

Treatment: *Punarnava* (*Boerhaavia diffusa*), especially its root is most effective in treating oedema. Punarnava mandura, a herbal recipe, is an iron preparation to which *punarnava* is added. It is usually available in Ayurvedic centres in the form of powder or pills. If there is constipation, it helps to relieve it and a certain amount of fluid goes out of the body through the stool. It improves the function of the kidneys and promotes urination.

Diet and regimen: Salt, fried foods and curd are strictly prohibited. Gourd, bitter gourds, plenty of ripe papaya (especially if constipated) are good. Excess fat, either of vegetable or of animal origin and particularly groundnuts are to be avoided. It is better not to sleep during the day. If there is fatigue, rest is advised but not sleep. As far as possible, sedentary habits must be avoided.

ᕙ Hysteria

Hysteria or *unmada* is a common emotional reaction, whereby the patient's distress is expressed in an exaggerated and dramatic form. Women outnumber men in this particular disease. Often

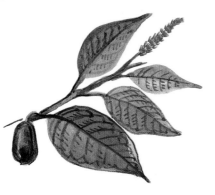

Haritaki *fruit is an effective cure for bronchial asthma.*

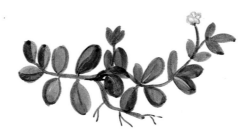

Brahmi *helps in calming the mind in hysteria.*

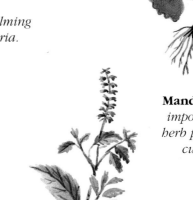

Mandukaparni *is an important medicinal herb prescribed for the cure of leprosy.*

Basil *juice regulates the heart.*

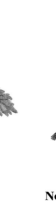

Katuki *is useful in liver cirrhosis.*

Neem *flowers are a prescribed diet in cervical spondylosis.*

Vasa *is very useful in curing chronic bronchitis.*

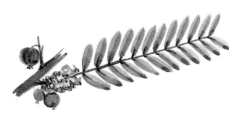

Amalaki *fruit, one of the richest sources of Vitamin C, is good for the heart as well as for asthmatic patients.*

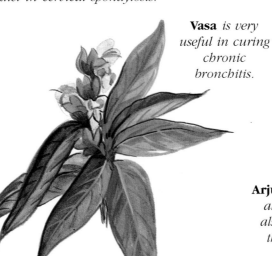

Arjuna, *good for the over-all health of the heart, also prevents clotting in the coronary arteries.*

children are also affected by it. Though the symptoms of hysteria are connected with neurotic or emotional factors, physically the patient may suffer from hyperacidity or heart burn, indigestion, or even an ulcer. Allergy, skin eruption or other types of organic and physical illness may be manifestations of psychosomatic disease.

Treatment: *Sarpagandha, brahmi (Centella asiatica), vacha (Acorus calamus)* and *shankhapushpi (Evolvulus alsinoides)* are used for treatment. They affect both the body and the mind. *Ashvagandha (Withania somnifera)*, an ingredient of Ashvagandharishta, a tonic, also gives relief.

Diet and regimen: Hot, spicy and fried food, as also pulses should be avoided. Almonds and almond oil are advised. One teaspoonful of almond oil, mixed with a cup of milk, taken before sleeping, helps to strengthen the nervous system. Mangoes, oranges, apples, peaches and bananas are also useful. A full night's sleep and an early morning walk help develop the will-power essential to overcome this disease.

❧ Sciatica

Sciatica or *gridhrasi* is a kind of nervous pain in the region of the buttocks, back of the thigh and the leg in which the sciatic nerve is present. Aggravation of vayu and physical strain are factors leading to its manifestation. Constipation often precipitates or aggravates an attack of sciatica.

Treatment: Eranda paka, an Ayurvedic mixture, helps sciatic patients who are constipated because it acts as a laxative. *Guggulu (Commiphora mukul)* is popularly used for the treatment of all pains of the nervous system and is an important ingredient in the drug Yogaraja guggulu. Saindhavadi taila, a medicinal oil, is useful for massage on the painful parts specially on the affected buttock from the top down. After hot fomentation with warmed rock salt tied in a linen cloth at bedtime, the buttock and leg should be covered with a warm cloth.

Diet and regimen: Pulses, beans and fried foods are strictly prohibited. Curd or anything sour, including sour fruits should be avoided. Saffron dissolved in warm milk is helpful. Gentle exercise of the leg is useful. Strenuous exercise including running and jumping is prohibited. Warm water baths are recommended. Swimming in moderately cold water is, however, considered to be very beneficial.

❧ Amoebic Dysentery

Amoebic dysentery or *pravahika* is an infection caused by a micro organism. According to Ayurveda, this organism is only a secondary factor.

Irregularity of diet, intake of heavy, indigestible food and emotional factors like worry, anxiety and anger are mainly responsible for the manifestation of this disease. In amoebic dysentery, frequent stools with mucus occur, invariably preceded by a gripping pain. There is loss of appetite and the patient feels excessively weak. In chronic cases, the

Lemon juice or just the fruit is an effective cure for amoebic dysentery.

liver is seriously affected and the patient loses a lot of weight.

Treatment: A decoction of the bark of kurchi or *kutaja* (*Holarrhena antidysenterica*) is used for treatment of dysentery. Constipation may also be present. The husk of flea seed or *isabgol* (*Plantago major*) should be taken at night with milk or butter-milk to counter this problem. In chronic dysentery, Rasaparpati, a preparation of mercury and sulphur, is popularly used.

Diet and regimen: The patient should avoid taking spices, chillies and fried food. Curd mixed with rice is beneficial, as also gruel. Vegetables and meat should be eaten as little as possible; if eaten at all, they should be in the form of soups. Sour and astringent tasting fruits like lemon, *amalaki*, pomegranate, banana (both ripe and green) are also useful.

Complete bed rest is essential specially in the acute stage of the attack. Avoid bathing as far as possible.

ॐ Liver Cirrhosis

Liver damage leads to chronic gastritis, morning sickness and constipation. Apart from loss of appetite, the patient loses weight because of defective metabolism. He may suffer from diarrhoea and flatulence and pain in the right upper portion of the abdomen where the liver is located. Slowly, the size of the liver increases and because of the pressure on the diaphragm, there is difficulty in breathing and cough. The liver tissue becomes fibrosed and shrinks in size causing obstruction in the veinous circulation and water accumulates in the abdomen.

Treatment: Cirrhosis of the liver generally occurs because of faulty diet and excessive intake of alcohol. It is imperative to give these up immediately. The *katuki* rhizome or root is medicinal in cirrhosis. Powdered *katuki* taken in a cup of warm water, acts as a purgative by stimulating the liver to produce more bile. The excretion of this bile in large quantities relieves the congestion in the liver and the tissues which have gone defunct start reviving.

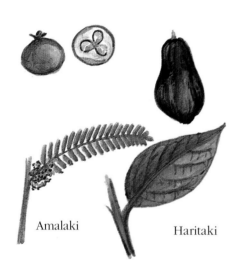

Amalaki

Haritaki

Amalaki *and* haritaki *are used in making Triphala powder, an important purgative.*

Katuki is an ingredient of a compound preparation called Arogyavardhini. It also contains copper which is a potent drug to revive the activity of different tissue cells.

Diet and regimen: Food which is difficult to digest, as well as oil, *ghee* and other such fats are to be avoided. Vegetables like bitter gourd are good. Milk containing a high percentage of fat is prohibited, though a small quantity of goat's and cow's milk is allowed. Curd should be avoided but butter-milk can be drunk. Garlic and a salt free diet are essential if there is accumulation of water in the abdomen. Fasting helps in promoting the function of the liver.

Sleeping during the day, riding a fast moving vehicle on an uneven surface, strenuous physical exercise are prohibited.

❧ Cervical Spondylosis

Cervical spondylosis or *griva sandhigata vata* is an osteo-arthritic type of spondylosis which frequently occurs in the cervical vertebrae. Factors like trauma, incorrect posture of the body, pressure while sleeping and excessive intake of sour food usually precipitate attacks of cervical spondylosis. Pain in the back of the neck, shoulder and arms, stiffness of the neck and even paraplegia occur due to this condition. The pain in the neck is generally aggravated by the movement of the spine. It is often associated with loss of memory and sleeplessness.

Treatment: The gum-resin *guggulu* is an important ingredient used in the preparation of Simhanada guggulu, a tonic, commonly used for the treatment of this condition. Usually hot water or hot milk is taken after a dose of this medicine. Since the bowels have to be cleared regularly, taking a purgative like Triphala powder (made of three medicinal herbs: *amalaki, haritaki, bibhitaki* or *Terminalia belerica*) at night is helpful. Fomentation on the neck vertebrae with about 500 gm of rock salt tied in a piece of cloth and heated in a frying pan till it becomes tolerably hot for half an hour everyday before sleeping is advised. Sometimes cervical spondylosis patients are unable to feel the quantum of heat, as they develop anaesthetic patches on the back, neck, shoulders and arms. Care should be taken to see that the cloth is not excessively hot.

Diet and regimen: Sour foods, particularly curd, are strictly prohibited, as are fried food and pulses. Bitter vegetables like *neem* (*Azadirachta indica*) flowers and bitter-gourd are very useful. Wheat is better than rice. Exposure to cold, a cold bath and any violent exercise of the neck muscles are very harmful. A comfortable posture should be maintained while reading or writing so that pressure is not put on the neck muscles. If the pain is acute, even an ordinary head bath is prohibited. A morning walk gives considerable relief to the patient; but if it is cold outside, the patient should always wrap a scarf around his neck.

❧ Diabetes

In Ayurveda, this is known as *madhumeha*. *Madhu* means honey and *meha* to pass out through the urine. Our modern life style is the prime cause of

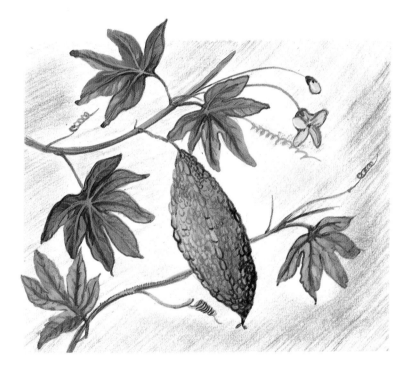

Bitter gourd is prescribed for patients of cervical spondylosis.

the disease. Excessively starchy diets, the manner in which we eat and drink, intake of tinned and preserved food, mental stress and strain, lack of exercise are responsible factors.

Treating diabetes means a strict regimen whereby sedentary habits are avoided and a certain amount of physical exercise is undertaken. Food which helps the action of the enzymes should be eaten. Most pungent and bitter foods work towards this. Thus, turmeric, bitter vegetables like bitter gourd and fenugreek are recommended. Honey, though a form of sugar, is not prohibited in diabetes. Collected from different types of flowers which may be astringent and bitter in taste, honey, if pure and natural, may cure diabetes. Honey from *neem* flowers is particularly useful.

Treatment: There are fourteen medicinal sources with anti-diabetic properties, preparations of which relieve the manifested signs and symptoms of diabetes, and also tries to curb the disease at its root. All these drugs primarily work at the site of origin of the disease. They directly affect the pancreas and liver. They provide the tissues of these glands with proper nourishment and help to tone them up. The pituitary gland at the base of the brain also gets rejuvenated and exercises better control over the liver, the pancreas, the suprarenal glands and the kidneys.

All these herbs act as a tonic on the nervous system in general, which in turn controls the secretion of insulin. Unlike insulin, they do not work as a replacement therapy, but reconstruct the body, activate and rejuvenate the body tissues and promote the production of insulin and utilisation of sugar by the tissues to produce energy. These herbs take long to act, but if taken for a prolonged period, the disease is eradicated. Some of these herbs produce a feeling of quick recovery from the disease, with symptoms like excessive hunger, urination, fatigue. The fall in blood-sugar level, however, takes a longer time.

The juice of the *bimbi's* (*Coccinia indica*) thick tuberous roots and its leaves and stems are used in treatment. The sap from the root of the gular fig tree or *udimbara* (*Ficus racemosa*) is useful. It acts as a very good tonic and simultaneously cures diabetes. If powdered fenugreek seeds processed in milk is taken for six months at a stretch, it also helps patients suffering from a very high blood sugar level. Bitter-gourd juice and mineral pitch (*shilajatu*) are highly recommended medicines.

Regimen: Sleeping during the day is strictly prohibited. Moderate exercise, especially Yoga is advisable.

❧ Rheumatism

Rheumatism or *amavata* is caused by the production and accumulation of a substance called *ama* in the body. *Ama* is produced by improper digestion as well as metabolism, and lodges itself in the joints and causes inflammation and pain. Usually persons with a constipative tendency and dietary irregularities are affected by *amavata*.

Treatment: Mahayogaraja guggulu and Simhanada guggulu, the medicines useful in this disease have the herb *guggulu* as their main constituent. If there is a constipative tendency Simhanada guggulu is more useful; otherwise, Mahayogaraja guggulu is better. Normally, a cup of warm water should be drunk after having the medicine. For weak and emaciated patients, a cup of milk is advised. The dose of this medicine should be slowly increased. These medicines have no toxic effects whatsoever, but the patient may, at times, feel slightly hot and in that case, the dosage should be reduced.

For the medicines to be really effective, constipation should be cured. Castor oil is considered to be the best purgative. *Haritaki* powder may be used as an alternative. Saindhavadi taila, a medicated oil, should be applied over the affected joints and rubbed gently.

Diet and regimen: Curd, anything sour, pulses (except *mung*) are prohibited. Fried and very cold food should be avoided as far as possible.

Sleep during the day is prohibited. Restricted physical exercise is allowed, but long, fast walks and any exercise involving violent movements of the affected joints should be avoided.

❧ Rheumatoid Arthritis

Rheumatoid arthritis begins by affecting the joints and which become swollen and painful and spreads to other parts of the body.

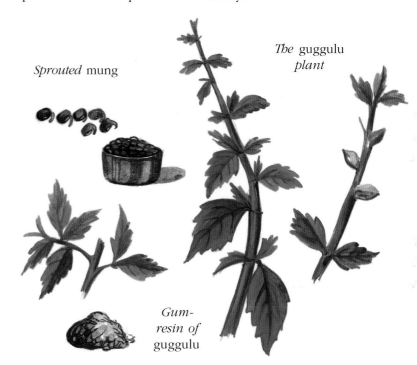

Sprouted mung

The guggulu *plant*

Gum-resin of guggulu

Sprouted mung is *the only kind of pulses allowed in the diet of a rheumatic patient. The gum-resin of* guggulu *is the most important ingredient used in medicines which cure rheumatism.*

Treatment: This disease may cause deformity if not treated immediately. In the initial stage,

Adding **cumin seeds** to the food during an attack of dystentery is beneficial.

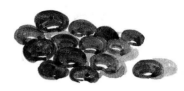

Mung. This pulse is good for the heart as well as rheumatic patients.

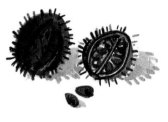

Castor seeds. Oil derived from them is an excellent purgative.

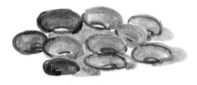

Masoor. This pulse too is good for the heart.

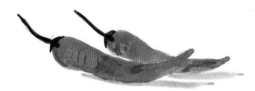

Chillies are usually asked to be avoided by Ayurvedic physicians as in most diseases, they are a harmful condiment.

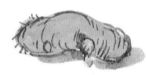

Turmeric powder mixed with warm water is an effective cure for bronchitis.

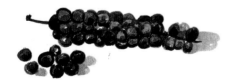

Black pepper is very useful in combating heart diseases.

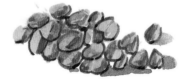

Fenugreek seeds help in curing diabetes.

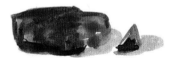

Asafoetida is good if taken when there is an attack of cough.

Mahayogaraja guggulu is useful. In winter, a larger dose is taken than in summer. A medicated oil, namely, Mahanarayana taila should be used for a gentle massage over the joints. In winter, it should be slightly warmed before use. In the beginning, this disease affects the small joints in fingers. Stiffness of the small muscles of the hands generally comes next and the fingers tend to get bent and ultimately become frozen. The infection then spreads towards the trunk involving the wrist joints, ankle joints, elbow joints, knee joints, shoulders, hips and jaws. If the bigger joints are affected then Brihadvata chintamani, another recipe of medicinal plants, is used. The dosage depends on the intensity of pain and duration of disease. Castor oil should be taken as a purgative every evening. Apart from its purgative effect, castor oil has a therapeutic effect on the patient's joints.

Diet and regimen: Anything sour including curd, pulses and preparations of pulses, fried food and constipating foods are to be shunned. Garlic and ginger are extremely useful. Five cloves of raw garlic should be taken daily, along with the day's food. Bitter vegetables like bitter-gourd, drumstick and *neem* flowers are advisable. Rice should be avoided.

Because of the inflammation, the patient is advised to restrict movement. But the joints should not remain immobilised, as this may result in permanent deformity. Light and gentle exercise is always needed. Exposure to cold winds or rain and cold water baths are to be avoided. A gap of about three hours should elapse between supper and bedtime.

❧ Migraine

Migraine or *anantavata* is a type of headache which is characterised by recurring paroxysmal attacks. Often only one side of the patient's head pains. Between the attacks, the patient feels perfectly well and leads a normal life. Sometimes the headache increases as the sun moves up in the sky, and the patient feels normal as the sun goes down. Excessive worry and anxiety is considered to be the primary cause of this type of headache. Exposing the head to the hot sun, cold wind or snow for a long time is one of the precipitating factors. Many patients suffering from migraine also suffer from sinusitis. Vomiting may accompany a severe attack. Between two attacks, the patient feels normal but a trace of heaviness in the head and congestion in the nose remains.

Treatment: Indigestion often precipitates attacks of this disease. In case of nausea, vomiting relieves indigestion and thus, the patient is relieved of headache. Even if there is no nausea, inducing vomiting by drinking 5-6 glasses of lukewarm water with a little salt or irritating the throat with a finger may help. Constipation is a constant and major complaint. A teaspoon of Triphala powder taken regularly at night with a cup of hot milk is a good antidote.

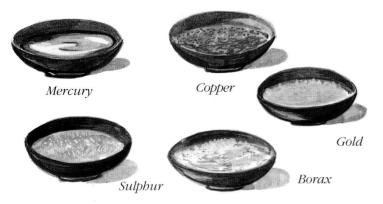

Mercury

Copper

Gold

Sulphur

Borax

Ingredients which constitute Suvarna sutashekhara, an important Ayurvedic drug for migraine.

Oleation or nasal inhalation of medicinal oils like Anu taila (made from sesame oil) or Shadbindu taila, both herbal oils, gives instant relief. The drug Suvarna sutashekhara is also used in treatment. It contains mercury, gold, copper, sulphur and borax in ash form. Godanti bhasma, a therapeutic mixture which is very cheap, is also used.

Diet and regimen: Fried, spicy foods are harmful. Curd and anything sour should be avoided.One must be free from indigestion, constipation, mental worries and anxieties. Exposure to excessive heat, cold and rain must be avoided.

✌ Hiccups

Hiccups or *hikka roga* is produced as a result of spasms of the glottis and diaphragm. Depending upon the doshas involved in the pathogenesis of the disease, different types of symptoms are manifested.

Treatment: Peacock feather ash mixed with honey is considered to be the best therapy for the condition. Eladi vati, which contains cardamom as an important ingredient, is also a popular tonic in this treatment. It is usually taken with honey.

Diet and regimen: Leftover cooked rice, tender radish, lemon, goat's milk and garlic is advisable. Fatty, heavy and cold food is not permitted. Rest is necessary. Natural urges should not be suppressed.

✌ Colic Pain

Colic pain or *shuta* is acute, paroxysmal abdominal pain. The pain may appear all of a sudden or gradually. Depending upon the causes, the pain can be of several types. The common causes of colic are appendicitis, gall-stone, kidney stone, intestinal spasm, duodenal and gastric ulcer and inflammation of the ovary or liver. Digestion and appetite are usually affected. The patient is constipated. The pain might spread to other parts of the body such as the scapular region, or the genital organs. There might be vomiting and nausea. Other symptoms vary depending upon the organ or part of the body affected. It is mainly caused by aggravation of vayu.

Treatment: To begin with, a mild purgative like castor oil or *isabgol* is taken. This removes constipation which alleviates vayu. Hingvashtaka churna (an easily available Ayurvedic recipe) which contains asafoetida as an important ingredient and Lasunadi vati containing garlic are generally used as medicines. Though this disease may automatically subside with little or no treatment, it may recur when there is any irregularity in eating habits or with psychological stress or strain. For permanent cure of this disease, a medicated *ghee*, Sukumara ghrita, made of *ghee* and castor oil, taken for a sufficiently long time even after the colic pain is over, is considered the best.

Diet and regimen: Food which has a drying effect on the body is prohibited. Pulses of all types, fried food, spices, chillies and anything sour are not allowed too. Milk, cheese, *ghee*, rice, wheat, *amalaki* and pomegranate are permitted.

Mental stress and strain, worry and anxiety are to be avoided. It is necessary to have sufficient rest and not remain hungry for long hours. Adequate sleep, especially an hour or so after lunch, may be helpful. Constipation leads to flatulence in the

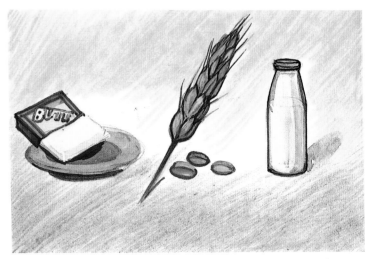

Cheese, wheat and milk are part of the prescribed diet for colic pain.

abdomen which precipitates or aggravates the attack of pain.

❧ Eczema

Eczema or *vichachika* means a 'boiling over' of the skin and is characterised by spontaneous eruptions.

It is primarily of two types, dry and wet. In the former, there is no secretion whereas in the latter, water may come out of the patches, either by scratching or without it.

Treatment: The eczema affected patch should be cleaned daily with warm water boiled with *neem* bark. After cleaning, the paste of the bark should be applied over it and allowed to dry. Paradadi malham, a concoction of many medicinal plants which contains mercury and sulphur among other items, should be applied three times daily. For internal administration, Shuddha gandhaka, a sulphur drug mixed with honey, is taken on an empty stomach. In chronic cases, Rasa manikya, an arsenic preparation can also be given. Paradadi malham and Rasa manikya should not be used in infant eczema as they are poisonous and may cause other complications.

Diet and regimen: Salt intake should be reduced, specially if taking Rasa manikya. Sour items including pickles and curd are strictly prohibited. Bitter gourd and *neem* flowers are very useful. Turmeric is perhaps the best as it can be applied externally over the eczematous patch and can be taken internally with milk. Nylons, terylenes and other synthetic fibres should be avoided as they inhibit evaporation of perspiration. The eczematous patches should be kept free from any tight clothing.

❧ Obesity

Obesity or *medoroga* is excessive accumulation of fat in the body. The most common areas where fat accumulates are the abdomen, breasts and buttocks. Excessive intake of fats and carbohydrates results in obesity. A lack of exercise helps accumulate fat in the body. Also, a lack of mental work aids the synthesis of fat from the carbohydrates taken through food. This fat, instead of being consumed, gets deposited in the body. The most common difficulty experienced because of excessive fat is breathlessness on even slight exertion. A serious type of asthma may develop. The function of the vital organs like the heart, liver and the kidneys may also be affected.

Treatment: Sedentary habits are to be countered. Persons working in offices should take a little walk after their meal. The gum resin extracted from *guggulu* is used in treatment. *Guggulu* is purified by a special process before it is administered internally. Compound preparations of *guggulu*: Navaka guggulu and Triphala guggulu can be taken as tablets.

Diet and regimen: *Haritaki* is very useful in this condition as it helps clear the bowels and works as a tonic. As far as possible, sweet and fatty foods, rice and potato which contain a lot of carbohydrates should be avoided. Among cereals, although, wheat is the best; barley and maize are also helpful. Bitter vegetables like bitter gourd, bitter varieties of drumstick are useful. Reasonable amounts of tea and coffee are allowed.

Sleeping during the day is not favourable though sleeping late at night and getting up early in the morning is very beneficial. Regular and adequate mental and physical exercise should be made a habit.

Home Remedies

ૐ Influenza

Description: Influenza is an infectious disease, marked by depression, distressing fever, acute catarrhal inflammation of the nose, larnyx and bronchi, neuralgic and muscular pains, gastro-intestinal disorders and nervous disturbances. It is caused by a virus and often occurs in epidemic form. It usually occurs during changes of season. Persons with a constipative tendency, and morbidity of the nasal mucous membrane or throat are more prone to this disease.

Remedies:

- Since the disease is generally associated with gastric disorder, long pepper is considered to be useful for its treatment. Half a teaspoonful of the powder of long pepper should be mixed with about two teaspoonfuls of honey and half a teaspoon of ginger juice. This may be given to the patient three times a day. If this mixture is given at the onset of fever, the patient's temperature can be arrested. It also promotes resistance against attacks of bronchitis and throat congestion.

- Basil leaves mixed with an equal quantity of dried ginger powder can be drunk in milk and sugar three to four times a day.

- A simple but very effective remedy is turmeric. One teaspoonful of turmeric powder or paste should be added to a cup of sweetened milk and taken three times a day. This induces an early recovery. It cures malaise and removes constipation, while keeping the lungs clear of phlegm and activating the liver.

Diet and regimen: After the onset of fever, it is better not to eat or eat very light meals. Barley water boiled with milk and sugar may be taken as also bread, biscuits, meat soup and vegetable soup. Garlic, either raw or fried with *ghee* or butter, is very useful. About ten cloves of garlic can be given to the patient. Green ginger may be added to the soup or vegetables. Heavy food like meat, chicken, fish and eggs, rice, wheat, *chapati* (a small, flat thin cake of coarse unleavened bread), fried food and sour items including curds are strictly prohibited during fever. Bananas, guavas and other sour fruits are allowed. Tea is not advisable, but coffee can be drunk in small quantities.

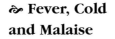

Turmeric plant

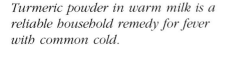

Turmeric powder in warm milk is a reliable household remedy for fever with common cold.

❧ Fever, Cold and Malaise

Fever with cold and malaise is a common ailment. It generally occurs during seasonal changes and exposure to rain as well as cold. The symptoms associated with these ailments are cough, a sore throat, sneezing, headache, watering of eyes, pain in the chest, loss of appetite and fatigue.

Remedies:
- One teaspoonful (5 gm) of turmeric powder can be taken three times a day mixed in a cup of warm milk.
- One teaspoonful (5 ml) of ginger juice three times a day with honey, may be taken.
- One teaspoonful of the powder of long pepper can be taken three times a day with honey.
- Tea prepared by adding the powder of ginger, black pepper and long pepper can be drunk three times per day.

Diet and regimen: Curd, sour food, cold drinks, heavy and fried food should be avoided. Garlic, ginger, black pepper and long pepper in food are useful. Rest is advised as also avoiding exposure to cold and rain.

❧ Cough

Cough is a symptom of several diseases affecting the chest and throat. It may be accompanied by sputum or it may be just a dry cough. It may be acute or chronic. Irritation and pain in the throat, spitting out large quantities of sputum which may be foul smelling; pain in the chest, back and abdomen; fever, loss of appetite, vomiting; difficulty in breathing; spitting of blood and loss of weight; headache, sneezing, giddiness and sleeplessness are symptoms associated with cough.

Remedies:

- For cough associated with spitting of sputum, slight pain in the chest and loss of appetite, juice, paste or powder of *vasa* (1 teaspoonful) with honey (1 teaspoonful) and ginger juice (½ teaspoonful) is advisable.
- For cough associated with irritation and pain in the throat, hot tea prepared with basil leaves, clove and ginger juice (½ teaspoonful) should be taken three times a day.
- For cough associated with fever, sneezing, headache and loss of appetite, half a teaspoonful of the powder of long pepper, black pepper and dry ginger (all three in equal quantities) may be taken with one teaspoonful of honey or a cup of warm milk three times a day.
- Hot fomentation of the chest with sand or rock salt tied in a piece of cloth is useful.
- Applying mustard oil on the chest and throat can help.

Diet and regimen: Curd, bananas, oranges, cold beverages and oily food are to be avoided. Garlic, ginger, turmeric, black pepper, cumin seeds, asafoetida and fenugreek seeds may be useful if taken in food. Drink only warm water. Do not sleep during the day, especially after eating. Avoid exposure to rain and cold and wear sufficient warm clothing. If there is constipation, take a mild laxative, i.e. one teaspoonful (5 gm) of *haritaki* powder before going to bed with warm water or warm milk.

❧ Headache

Headache can occur in several diseases. It can be

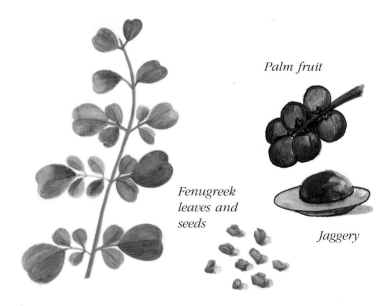

Palm fruit

Fenugreek leaves and seeds

Jaggery

Fenugreek seeds can cure cough. Jaggery obtained from palm fruit has many remedial properties, one of them is curing headache.

in any part of the head. It may occur occasionally or may persist. It may also increase as the day begins and diminish at sunset. Defective eyesight may give rise to headache.

Remedies:

- For headache associated with constipation, take one teaspoonful (5 gm) of *haritaki* powder with hot water or hot milk at bedtime.
- One teaspoonful (5 gm) of the powder of long pepper could be taken three times per day with water, preferably by adding one teaspoonful of jaggery.
- For headache associated with sore throat and cold, take one teaspoonful of ginger juice with honey three times a day.

  Diet and regimen: Avoid fried food and spices.

✎ Vomiting

Vomiting is generally caused by an infection in the stomach or by eating and drinking contaminated or stale food and drinks. It also occurs in early pregnancy. Pain in the abdomen, diarrhoea, constipation and fever accompanies vomiting. Severe vomiting may lead to dehydration, especially in children.

Remedies:

- One teaspoonful (5 ml) of lemon juice three times a day with a pinch of salt can curb vomiting.
- One teaspoonful (5 gm) of cardamom powder three times a day with hot water is helpful too.

- For vomiting with abdominal pain, one teaspoonful of lemon juice with one gram of asafoetida powder is helpful. Also one teaspoonful (2.5 gm) of nutmeg powder with butter-milk or curd is an effective cure.
- For vomiting with fever, take one teaspoonful (5 ml) of lemon juice and half a teaspoonful (2.5 ml) of ginger juice with a pinch of salt.

✎ Constipation

A person who complains of constipation passes dry and hard stools less frequently than once a day. Constipation may be acute, developing suddenly or long standing (chronic). Acute constipation may be symptomatic of a more serious illness. Such cases should be referred to the hospital immediately. Constipation may also occur following an attack of diarrhoea or the day after taking a purgative. Constipation is common in old people and during pregnancy. Constipation in children is due to faulty dietary habits. Abdominal discomfort and pain, loss of appetite and headache are commonly associated with constipation.

Remedies:

- For constipation in babies, one gram of *isabgol* husk, three times a day, with warm milk or warm water and a pinch of sugar may be given.

- For constipation in pregnant women, two teaspoonfuls (10 gm) of *isabgol* husk, twice daily with warm milk or warm water can be taken.
- For constipation in adults, one teaspoonful (5 gm) of *haritaki* powder or two teaspoonfuls (10 gm) of *isabgol* husk at bedtime with hot water or hot milk is advised. The former is more powerful than the latter.
- For constipation associated with pain in the abdomen, one teaspoonful (5 gm) of *haritaki* powder and one gram of ginger mixed together, is effective. If vomiting and abdominal pain accompanies constipation, a doctor should be consulted.

Diet and regimen: Less meat, eggs and fried food should be eaten. Instead, the diet should contain more leafy vegetables and fruits. The common cause of constipation is carelessness in not going to the toilet especially when there is an urge for defecation.

❧ Indigestion

This is generally caused by overeating, irregular eating habits and by eating heavy, fried, infected and contaminated food. Pain in the abdomen, burning sensation in the chest, acid eructations, loss of appetite, nausea, vomiting and diarrhoea are normally associated with indigestion.

Remedies:
- Chewing a piece of ginger (about 2 gm) with a pinch of salt, five minutes before a meal prevents and cures indigestion.

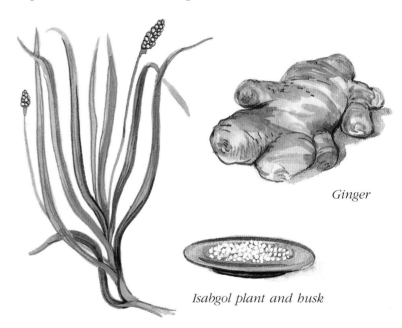

Ginger

Isabgol plant and husk

Isabgol husk in warm water is the most effective cure for constipation. Chewing a piece of ginger before eating prevents and cures indigestion.

- Chewing 2 gm of *haritaki* pulp with jaggery five minutes before a meal also helps .
- Taking one teaspoonful of ginger juice with an

equal quantity of lemon juice and a pinch of salt twice a day is useful.

- One teaspoonful of the powder, paste or juice of nutgrass or *Cyperus rotundus* may be taken three times a day. Honey or sugar may be added to this.

Diet and regimen: Heavy and fried foods are to be strictly avoided.

❧ Diarrhoea

Passing of frequent loose stools is called diarrhoea. It could be caused by food and drinks contaminated by disease-causing germs or eggs of worms. Adults, old people and small babies are equally affected by this ailment. But small babies need extra care. Vomiting, pain in the abdomen, loss of appetite and disturbed sleep are some common symptoms of diarrhoea. Serious types of diarrhoea may lead to dehydration, particularly in babies.

Remedies:
- For diarrhoea in adults and old persons: take one teaspoonful (5 gm) of a paste or powder prepared by mixing equal amounts of *bael* fruit and nutmeg seeds, three times a day. If there is blood in the stool, the juice of a medium-sized pomegranate should also be taken.

- For diarrhoea with vomiting, take the above-mentioned drugs with 1 gm of cardamom powder or one teaspoonful of lemon juice with salt.
- For diarrhoea with pain in the abdomen or loss of appetite, the same drug preparation should be taken with 1 gm of asafoetida powder.
- For diarrhoea where dehydration sets in early, take 10 gm of jaggery and 2 gm of salt in a cup of water (about 250 ml) and mix well. Drink this a little at a time.
- For chronic diarrhoea, take one teaspoonful (5 gm) of cumin powder three times a day with water. Sugar or honey may be added.

These remedies should bring relief within twenty four hours. If not, a doctor must be consulted.

Diet and regimen: Avoid all hard-to-digest fatty foods. Yoghurt or curd is very useful during a diahorreal attack as also a piece of hard toast without butter. Rest and adequate sleep is essential.

❧ Infantile Diarrhoea

Intake of stale milk or infection in the alimentary tract causes diarrhoea in children. If the child is fed on breast milk, the digestive capacity of the mother also affects the digestion of the milk by the child. Along with diarrhoea, the child may even start vomiting and there may be a sharp pain in the stomach. The stool may be liquid and foul-smelling, and it may be greenish or yellowish in colour. Diarrhoea is common when a child is teething.

Remedy: If diarrhoea is very intense and there is too much vomiting, 65 mg of nutmeg powder should be given to the child four times a day, mixed with honey.

Diet and regimen: Milk containing a high percentage of fat should not be given. If the mother is suffering from indigestion, she should also be treated if she is feeding the child.

✍ Dysentery

Frequent stools (often loose) with mucus, associated with a shooting pain in the abdomen characterize dysentery. It is caused by drinking infected water and eating contaminated food. Pain in the abdomen, loss of appetite, abdominal distension, fatigue and disturbed sleep are common symptoms. Occasionally blood may appear along with mucus in the stool.

Remedies:

- One teaspoonful (5 gm) of the powder of kurchi bark thrice a day with butter-milk or two tablespoonfuls (30 ml) of kurchi bark powder thrice a day with sugar, jaggery or honey is useful.

- *Isabgol* husk, two teaspoonfuls three times a day with curd or butter-milk can curb dysentery.

- For dysentery with a pronounced gripping pain, take one teaspoonful (5 gm) of *haritaki* powder twice daily with hot water.

- For dysentery with loss of appetite, take one teaspoonful of ginger powder or ginger juice (5 ml) three times per day with honey.

- For dysentery with very loose stool, take one teaspoonful of cumin seed powder with water.

Diet and regimen: Eating light meals, avoiding fried food, lentils, milk, curd and butter-milk are very useful. Adding salt and powdered cumin seeds to the food helps.

✍ Eye Discharge

Eye discharge occurs due to an infection or the entry of a foreign body in the eye. Red eyes, itching, burning sensation, watering, difficulty in vision, pain in the eyes, fever, headache, or a sore throat are associated symptoms.

Remedies:

- The eyes must be cleaned several times a day with cotton wool soaked in boiled lukewarm water. While boiling, add a teaspoonful of turmeric powder to 250 ml of water and boil for ten minutes. Strain and use the water to wash the eyes.

- One teaspoonful of turmeric powder or the

powder of the gum resin *guggulu* may be taken thrice a day with a cup of warm milk.

- One teaspoonful (5 gm) of *haritaki* powder can be taken at night with hot water.

Diet and regimen: Avoid yoghurts, exposure to cold, rain and bright light.

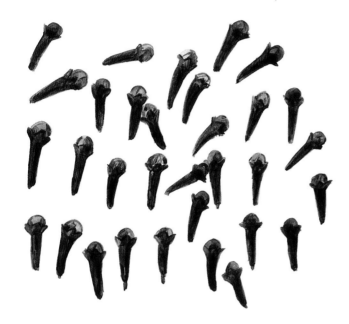

Applying clove oil is a very effective cure for toothache.

❧ Earache

Pain in the ear is usually caused by an infection in the ear or throat or by the intrusion of a foreign body inside the ear. Fever, sore throat, difficulty in hearing, discharge from the ear and giddiness are associated with earache. If the earache persists for over twenty-four hours, a doctor should be consulted.

Remedies:

- For earache associated with discharge from the ear, the ear should be cleaned gently using a clean piece of cotton wool swab.
- Boil almond oil with one teaspoonful of garlic juice. Strain and allow it to cool. When lukewarm, apply a few drops to the ear.
- Hot fomentation with sand or salt is useful.

Diet and regimens: Curd and sour food should be avoided, as also exposure to cold or rain.

❧ Toothache

Toothache is a common complaint, especially for people who do not take proper care of teeth. Inflammation of gums, bleeding from gums and headache are symptoms generally associated with this.

Remedies:

- Applying clove oil over the affected tooth.
- Chewing a few cloves with the affected teeth.
- Keeping asafoetida powder over the affected teeth.
- Washing the mouth with warm saline water in regular intervals.

Diet and regimen: Curd, sour and sweet things should be avoided. If unable to chew, a liquid diet is preferable. Garlic is also useful.

✎ Joint Pains

Joint pains may be caused by strain or injury or they may be a symptom of a disease. Chronic disease of a joint may lead to deformity. One or several joints may be affected simultaneously. Joint pains often occur in old persons. Red, hot, swollen or tender joints, and fever are often associated with joint pains.

Remedies:

- Six teaspoonfuls of a decoction of the root bark of castor plant may be taken three times a day.
- One teaspoonful (5 gm) of gum resin powder taken three times a day with any hot drink can help.
- If joints are swollen, red, hot and tender, keep a hot water bottle of the warm paste of castor root on the affected parts or apply lukewarm castor oil. Castor leaves smeared with a little castor oil and warmed by heating, may be placed over the affected joints.
- Five drops of castor oil in a cup of warm milk can be taken three to four times a day. Cardamom powder and sugar may be added to this mixture.

Warning: A child with severe pain in several joints and fever who shows no improvement after two days of treatment, should be taken to the nearest health centre or hospital.

Diet and regimen: Curd, sour food and alcoholic drinks are to be avoided. Garlic and ginger are useful. Avoid being out in the cold and rain. Take hot water baths (in winter) and drink hot water.

✎ Painful Menstruation

Pain usually occurs before the onset of menstruation or it may continue during the menstrual period. Pain in the back, thighs, lower abdomen, nausea,

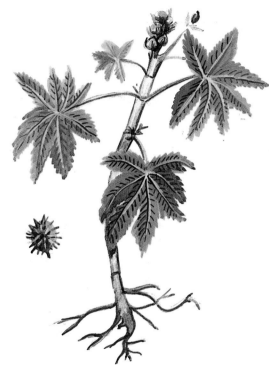

Castor leaves smeared with castor oil help mitigate joint pains.

headache, sleeplessness, vomiting and constipation are common symptoms associated with this.

Remedies:

- Hot fomentation may be given to the lower abdomen.
- Taking one teaspoonful of the powder of *haritaki* with hot water before going to bed is useful.
- Taking three cloves of garlic cut into small pieces, three times a day with hot water is advisable.
- One teaspoonful (5 gm) of fenugreek powder, may be taken three times a day with hot milk or hot water.

Diet and regimen: Heavy and fried food should be avoided. Rest and protection from cold and rain will help.

❧ Sprains

Sprains are caused by joints being twisted by a fall while running and jumping or if the foot falls accidentally on an uneven surface. Swelling and pain in the joints are common symptoms associated with sprains.

Remedies:

- Hot fomentation with sand or salt.
- Applying ginger paste over the affected joints and covering with a bandage.
- One teaspoonful (5 gm) of turmeric powder with any hot drink three times per day.

Warning: This treatment should be carried on for one week. If there is no relief, a doctor should be consulted.

Diet and regimen: Curd and sour food should be avoided. The affected part must be given sufficient rest.

❧ Cramps

An involuntary and painful contraction of a voluntary muscle or a group of muscles is known as cramps. Exercising in excess of one's capacity, indulgence in dry and rough food and taking harmful medicines may result in an attack. Cramps are also caused as symptoms of various other diseases.

Remedy: Massage is the best therapy. A medicated oil like Mahanarayana taila should be warmed in water and rubbed all over the body. Those who get cramps frequently can even use ordinary sesame oil and massage themselves before bathing. To relieve constipation, castor oil can be taken in an appropriate dose depending upon the constitution of the individual.

Diet and regimen: Foods like pulses are not advisable in cramps. Sufficient quantities of sweet and sour things, garlic and asafoetida are usually prescribed. Regular massage and exercise are useful, as also protection against cold winds and rain. Late nights, suppression of natural urges, worry, anxiety and anger should be avoided. Sleeping during the day is not advisable.

Ayurveda also prescribes certain remedies for serious epidemic as well as chronic ailments like malaria, measles, tubercolosis and tonsillitis. These cures can be tried out if the disease is in its early stages as they do not have any toxic side-effects.

✍ Malaria

Malaria, which is transmitted by the female anopheles mosquito, causes periodic fever, enlargement of the spleen and anaemia. The tonic Sudarshana churan which contains the herb *chirayata* (*Swertia chirata*) is generally used in treatment, as also *guduchi* (*Tinospora codiofoilia*) juice mixed with honey. Soups, barley water and milk should form the bulk of the patient's diet.

✍ Measles

Measles is a highly infectious disease characterized by catarrah of the respiratory passages and a widespread eruption on the skin. Powdered coral or Pravala pishti mixed with honey is recommended both for the prevention and cure of measles. The patient should be on a spartan diet of barley gruel and fruit juice.

✍ Tubercolosis

In Ayurveda, tubercolosis is said to be primarily caused due to a vitiation of the doshas and bacilli are considered to be secondary factors. *Vasa* is commonly suggested in the treatment of this disease. Dry fruits, almond oil, Chyavanaprasha and milk boiled with garlic are supposed to bring relief.

✍ Tonsillitis

Tonsillitis usually occurs in young children and is associated with fever and attacks of cold and cough. The tonsils in the throat become red and swollen and there is difficulty in swallowing. It is best to keep the neck as warm as possible. Daily gargles with rock salt and acacia or *babula* (*Acacia arabica*) bark gives relief to the pain. Dry, heavy or sour food should be avoided whereas meat soups, pulses and fenugreek are good for this condition.

Measures for Good Health

---- * ----

Maintaining good health and treatment of disease are two sides of the same coin. The food, drugs and regimen that Ayurveda prescribes for both are similar. The components are the same: they are all found in nature. Equal importance is given to the kind of food to be taken as to the drugs prescribed. Each reinforces the other and both act in similar ways to restore or maintain the equilibrium of the doshas in the body.

Regimen for the Day (Dinacharya)

Traditionally, a person should wake up before dawn when it is

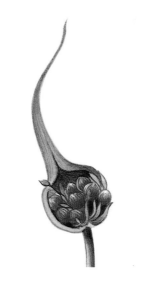

Yoga destroys despair; it is only for the moderate in eating and resting, in sleeping and working.

. . . The Bhagvad Gita

calm and quiet, the air is free from pollutants and there is time to pray or to meditate. There is also time enough to plan the day's work. After getting out of bed one should wash one's face with water—lukewarm or cold, according to the season. While gently splashing water over the eyes, it helps if one keeps one's mouth full of water. This helps exercise the eye-muscles. The eyes should be kept wide open while splashing water over them.

After this the teeth should be brushed. In India, twigs of the *neem* tree and others are used for brushing the teeth. The *neem* twig is chewed at the top while brushing. Herbal tooth powders and paste are also available. Along with brushing the teeth, scraping the tongue is also highly recommended. Again, this helps the eye muscles and therefore strengthens eyesight. Tongue scrapers should be made of gold, silver, copper, tin or brass. They should be curved and should have smooth edges.

After washing and cleaning one's face, it is always advisable to drink a glass of cold water. This is prescribed for all days in all seasons unless one has a cold, a cough or a sore throat. The importance of drinking a glass of water in the morning cannot be overemphasized for it helps in the excretory process. Drinking a cup of tea in the morning only produces pressure and stimulates the intestines to start the movement for evacuation of waste. It is like a reflex action which is different from the effect produced by drinking a glass of water. Hot tea stimulates the intestines so strongly that the effect loses its significance after some days leading to constipation. The caffeine content in tea or coffee also produces some adverse effects on the intestines. A glass of water, on the other hand, is excellent for the peristalsis of the intestines.

Evacuation of stool early in the morning should become a regular habit and a glass of cold water helps overcome any problems caused by indigestion and inadequate sleep if the previous night's meal has not been assimilated properly. Worry, anxiety, a short temper, over-sensitivity or anger cause a lot of wind to form in the stomach which gets accumulated in the intestines at night. Fried food and certain 'heavy' lentils cause flatulence as also the absence of an adequate

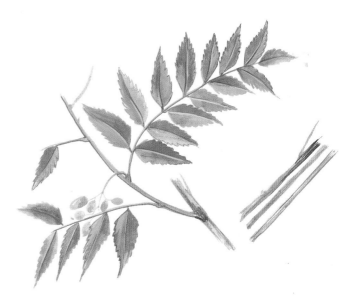

Neem *leaves and twigs. Brushing one's teeth with* neem *twigs is an ancient Indian practice as the medicinal properties of* neem *are manifold.*

quantity of leafy vegetables and fruit in one's diet. Flatulence causes obstruction and irregularity in bowel movements Very often this incomplete metabolic process leads to loss of appetite, indigestion, headache, fatigue and even sleeplessness. Excessive flatulence can also put pressure on the heart and cause palpitation. Proper food, drink and sleep are therefore of primary importance.

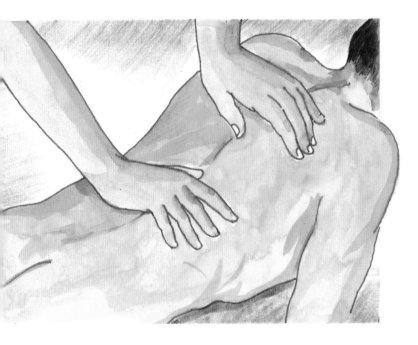

Oil massage invigorates the skin, tones up the nervous system and helps overcome fatigue.

❧ The Use of Oil

The use of oils in therapies can be of two kinds—internal and external. Oil massage for the body is an essential part of the daily routine in most parts of India. The oils used for this purpose are generally mustard oil, sesame oil and coconut oil. Massage with mustard oil, particularly in winter, is characteristic of the north of India while sesame oil is used in the south. Coconut oil is generally used for massaging the scalp and for luxuriant hair growth.

A good oil massage slows down the ageing process. It keeps the skin moisturized and shiny. It helps to overcome fatigue, tones up the nervous system, promotes eyesight and nourishes the body by opening the pores of the skin. A good oil massage followed by a bath helps one to sleep well and feel rested. Applying oil (sesame oil or coconut oil preferably) on the head quite regularly is a good way to prevent headaches, premature baldness and greying of hair and to prevent hair from falling. Massaging the body with oil is also somewhat like oiling a machine. It keeps it in shape. It strengthens and maintains the body and relaxes the muscles. It smoothens the skin and removes roughness and dryness, prevents susceptibility to vata-aggravated diseases and relieves exhaustion and the effects of exertion. It alleviates the effects of strenuous physical exercise and even of injuries.

Sesame oil has several excellent properties. It can be used for gargling, it effectively strengthens the jaws, gives depth to the voice, and a fuller look to the face, provides excellent gustatory sensation and increases appetite. Regular gargles with this oil prevent dryness in the throat and cracked lips, while massaging the gums with this oil strengthens them and prevents caries. The teeth become strong and less prone to disease.

Nasal inhalation with Anu taila during all the three seasons—the rainy season, autumn and spring—is an extremely useful practice with numerous benefits. Habitual nasal therapy according to the prescribed method helps keep the eyes, nose and ears healthy, restores and strengthens hair, prevents greying. Inhalation therapy also helps cure diseases such as torticolis, headache, facial paralysis, lockjaw, rhinitis, hemicrania and tremors of the head. It gives strength to the veins, joints, ligaments and tendons of the head and neck. The voice becomes stable and sweet and the face fills out. All the sense organs are regulated. Signs of age such as grey hair are not manifested. Oil used as ear-drops prevents deafness and other diseases of the ear.

Massaging the soles of the feet with oil cures roughness, immobility, dryness, fatigue and numbness. The feet become strong and steady and eyesight is improved because the eye muscles are strengthened through this. Regular oil massage of the feet helps prevent sciatica, cracks in the feet, and constriction of vessels and ligaments.

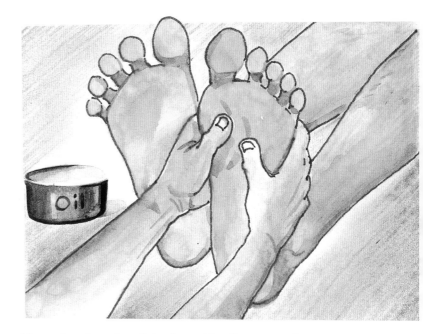

Massaging the soles of the feet with oil removes dryness, cracks and prevents sciatica.

Oleation relieves drowsiness and itching. It also eliminates unpleasant body odours because of perspiration.

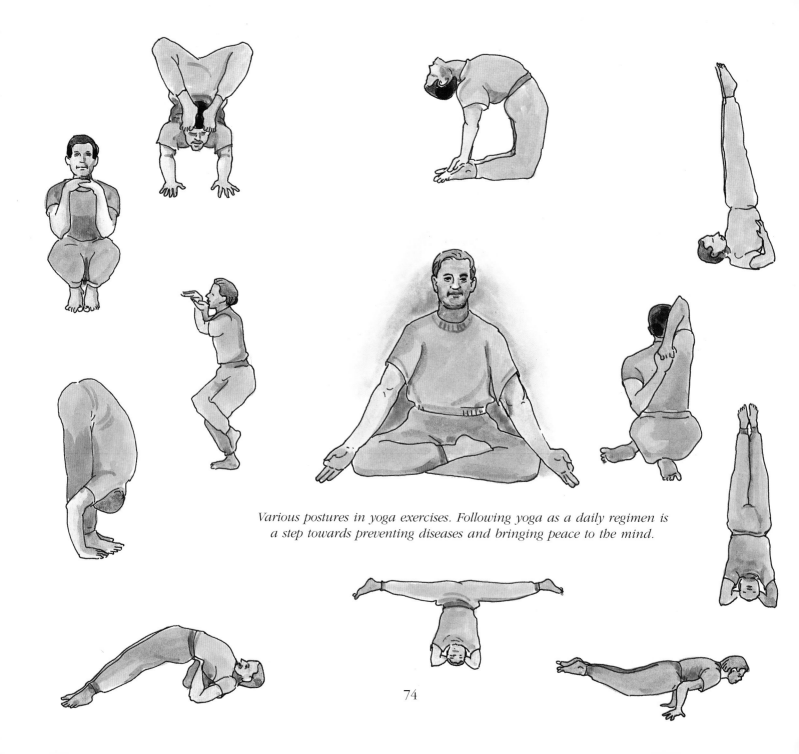

*Various postures in yoga exercises. Following yoga as a daily regimen is
a step towards preventing diseases and bringing peace to the mind.*

74

ஃ Exercise

Exercise, to be useful and productive, must be done with moderation. Physical exercise in excess causes exertion, exhaustion, consumption, thirst, bleeding from various parts of the body, acute form of dyspnoea, cough, fever and vomiting. On the other hand, if exercise is done correctly, there will be perspiration, enhanced respiration, a feeling of lightness, and proper functioning of the heart and other organs of the body. It also builds resistance and alleviates doshas especially kapha. It stimulates the power of digestion. Ayurveda does not recommend exercise while laughing, talking or walking or during sex. Exercise should be done in a relaxed manner, not on a full stomach, nor when one is tired. Rest after exercise is essential. Yoga is an excellent form of exercise helping the body, mind and soul.

A bath in the morning is not just refreshing but a sexual stimulant. It enhances stability in the body and gives it strength. Above all, it helps remove fatigue, dirt and perspiration. Generally, warm baths should be taken in winter or during the rains. Cold baths are better in warm weather. Hair and scalp should be washed with cold water. Wearing clean clothes adds to one's appearance and personal hygiene. Clean apparel inspires self-confidence. Enhancing one's looks and providing a well-groomed appearance can also be achieved by trimming one's hair and beard (for men), combing one's hair, keeping the finger-nails trimmed and clean. Longevity, cleanliness and beauty help in maintaining physical and mental well-being.

Proper and comfortable shoes preserve the skin of the feet. It protects the feet from contact with germs, disease-carrying bacteria and from the attacks of reptiles and other creatures.

ஃ Food

Food, an important factor in the maintenance of good health, should be eaten in proper quantities, depending upon the power of digestion and the metabolism of the individual. The right quantity of food is the amount which, without disturbing the equilibrium of tissues and doshas of the body, gets digested as well as metabolised in proper time. The power of digestion varies with individual metabolisms.

In Ayurveda, food is characterised as light or heavy. Food which is light is rich in the qualities of air and fire. Those dominated by earth and water are heavy. Light food stimulates appetite and is considered less harmful even if eaten in excess of the prescribed quantity. On the other hand, food which is heavy suppresses appetite and is exceedingly harmful if taken in excess unless the power of digestion and metabolism are greatly reinforced by physical exercise. If the food is heavy, only three-fourths or half of the stomach should be filled. Even in the case of light food, excessive intake is not conducive to the processes of digestion and metabolism.

Regimen for the Night (Ratricharya)

Proper sleep endows an individual with nourishment, strength, virility, knowledge, longevity and happiness. On the other hand, improper sleep causes misery, emaciation, weakness, sterility, and even early death. Untimely and excessive sleep as well as prolonged vigil take away both happiness and longevity.

Depending upon the causative factors, there are seven types of sleep: (1) sleep caused by lethargy, (2) sleep caused by the vitiation of kapha, (3) sleep caused by mental exertion, (4) sleep caused by physical exhaustion, (5) exotic type of sleep (*agantuka*) which is caused by artificial means like sedatives, (6) sleep caused by diseases, (7) sleep caused by nightfall when the body naturally demands sleep or physiological sleep.

It is not advisable to sleep during the day in seasons other than summer. Doing so causes vitiation of kapha and pitta. Obese people who are used to unctuous substances, those with a pitta constitution, those suffering from diseases due to the vitiation of kapha and those suffering from artificial poisoning (which happens when substances which are incompatible are mixed and consumed either deliberately or inadvertently; honey in hot water can act as a poison) should never sleep during the day. This could lead to liver problems, headache, heaviness of the body, fever, loss of digestive power, oedema, anorexia, nausea, urticaria, eruption, abscess, drowsiness, coughing, diseases of the throat, impairment of memory and intelligence, obstruction of the circulatory channels of the body and weakness of sensory and motor organs.

Sleeping during the day in all seasons is permitted for those who are exhausted by singing, studying, alcoholic drinks, sex, elimination therapy, carrying heavy weights, walking long distances; those suffering from diarrhoea, colic pain, dyspnoea, insanity; those who are too old, too young, weak and emaciated; those injured by fall and assault; those exhausted by a journey, vigil, anger, grief and fear. In summer, nights become shorter and vata gets aggravated in the body due to the absorption of fluid because of perspiration.

Therefore, during this season, sleep during the day is allowed for all.

❧ Causes of Sleeplessness

Elimination of doshas from the body through purgation and emesis; fear, anxiety, anger, smoke, physical exercise, excessive bleeding, fasting, uncomfortable beds go a long way towards overcoming sleep. The above-mentioned factors along with overwork, old age, diseases, specially those due to the vitiation of vata (like colic pain) are known to cause sleeplessness even in normal individuals.

❧ Measures to Induce Sleep

Sleep may be induced by massages, unction, baths, drinking meat soup, eating rice with curd, drinking milk and alcohol, giving the mind rest, peace and happiness and hearing soft pleasant music, applying soothing ointments to the eyes, head and face, having a comfortable bed and home and going to bed at an appropriate hour. There should be a sufficient gap between dinner and retiring for bed. This will aid the digestive process which in turn will result in good sleep. Food should, as far as possible, be light and easily digestible. Curd should be strictly avoided at night. Though good for health, curd has a negative effect on the channels of circulation when taken at night and obstructs them. It is specially unsuitable for patients who are suffering from asthma, bronchitis and rheumatism.

❧ Sex

One should not indulge in excessive sex. Sex should be avoided if there is no privacy, or if under pressure of the urge to micturate, after exertion, after physical exercise, while fasting, and if exhausted. A glass of milk should be taken before and after the sexual act.

❧ Natural Urges

The living body has some natural urges. They are the urge to urinate, to defecate, to have sexual intercourse, pass wind, for vomiting, sneezing, yawning, hunger, thirst, tears, and sleep. Inhibition of these natural urges leads to many complications. These complications affect digestion and metabolism which in turn can lead to several kinds of ailments. Therefore, in order to be able to sleep enough at night, it is essential to see that the body's natural urges are never curbed.

Therapy for Old People

The philosophy behind Ayurveda is to enable the individual to live his full span of life as a useful and productive member of society. By prescribing various diets and regimens along with therapies, Ayurveda aims to help the individual towards this end. Specialized therapies such as garlic and rejuvenation therapies have been touched upon in brief to show the scope of this complex system of medicine that heals and preserves at the same time.

❧ Rejuvenation Therapy

The average life span of an individual has increased in present times due to better quality of medical help and improved nutrition. Therefore, the number of old people in society has gone up. Rejuvenation or *rasayana* therapy, prescribed in Ayurveda, is meant to help improve the lives of old people. Charaka, while defining the scope of this therapy, states that through it, the individual is endowed with longevity; memory; intellect; positive health; youthfulness; excellent complexion, voice, strength of the sensory and motor organs and lustre. Instead of a society of old and invalid people, it aims at creating a society of aged people with youthful vigour—both physical and mental. Rejuvenation therapy aims at keeping the enzymes in the tissues cells in their normal functioning condition. These cells are revitalised and their composition is changed. Tranquility of the mind is promoted and the nerves as well as bones kept in good condition. This prevents the process of ageing and makes the individual free from any disease even in his advanced years. He is able to see as clearly as before and maintain his hearing abilities, as also the glow on his face and the colour of his skin. The sooner the therapy is administered to the individual the better. As a person grows older, this therapy becomes ineffective.

For rejuvenation, many drugs are described in Ayurvedic classics, and prescribed by Ayurvedic physicians. The most important ones are *amalaki, bibhitaki, haritaki, guduchi* and *brahmi*. Drugs of mineral origin like mercury, sulphur, gold and mineral pitch or bitumen are also extensively used for the purpose of rejuvenation. These drugs are detoxicated and assimilated before they are used. The mode of administration, the method of preparation, the dosage, the diet and the precautions to be taken while administering these drugs, vary from drug to drug. Normally, they

Facing page: *Different kinds of garlic used in garlic therapy. Garlic therapy is a type of rejuvenation therapy for old people which involves a complex and intense process of treatment and aftercare.*

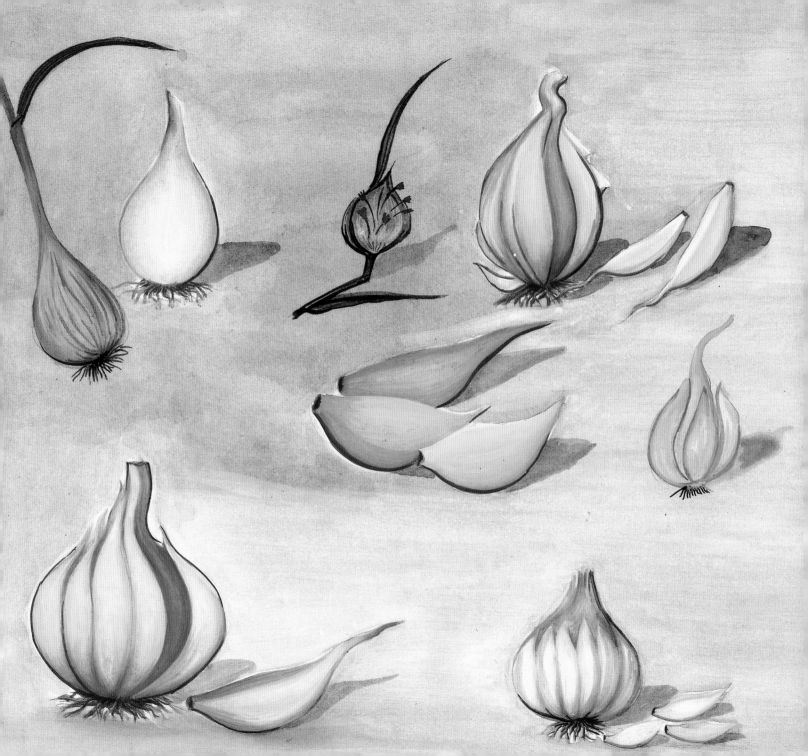

require the supervision of experts. To obtain the desired effect, the therapy should be followed for a considerable amount of time. The duration of this therapy depends on the age and other physical and psychological conditions of the individual.

There are many pharmaceutical processes to make these drugs palatable. The most common tonic used by Ayurvedic physicians is Chyavanaprasha. Ayurvedic physicians consider Chyavanaprasha more a food than a medicine. The dosage of this medicine has to be increased gradually. This medicine is absolutely non-toxic. But, at times, it suppresses the power of digestion, if the dose is increased all of a sudden.

ॐ Garlic Therapy

There are more than forty-five varieties of garlic which are used as medicine in several parts of the globe from Siberia to the tropical climes of India. Despite differences in colour and taste, they all have the characteristic odour of garlic. Its therapeutic properties are undisputed but Indian texts on religious rites categorize it as food that rouses passion and emotion or *rajsic* food. Hence, it is taboo for brahmins and those engaged in spiritual practices.

Garlic therapy or *rasona kalpa* which is a rejuvenation therapy can be administered only to persons who are physically strong and whose systems of digestion and metabolism are powerful. It should be administered only in certain seasons, according to the individual constitution of the person receiving the treatment. Ayurvedic texts are also emphatic in indicating the kinds of individuals (including children) who are not fit to receive this therapy. The list of such persons is fairly long and detailed.

For a long term effect and especially for rejuvenation, a large quantity of garlic has to be used which most people cannot tolerate. The procedure is therefore very gradual where due care is given to indications and contraindications. The plant has to be gathered in a specific manner and it has to be mixed with other drugs before administration. The dosage, the preparation of the patient, the processing of the drug and its administration are all part of a highly complex system which involves the patient and the physician in a protracted process of therapy and aftercare. Rejuvenation therapies likewise are not for everyone. These therapies can be administered only to persons who possess certain qualities that go to make a 'good' individual whose conduct and bearing in all respects make him or her an asset to society.

Glossary

———— * ————

Adhibhautika	Diseases which originate from external physical factors like germs and accidents.
Adhidaiveka	Diseases caused due to seasonal, planetary and providential influences.
Adhyatmika	Diseases which originate from the human body, including psychosomatic ones.
Adisthana	Site of manifestation of a disease.
Agantuka	Strange, exotic
Agni	Fire, one of the five elements that make up the universe; also refers to the 13 enzymes of the body.
Agnivesha	Sage Atreya's disciple who wrote the *Agnivesha Samhita.*
Agnivesha Samhita	Ancient Ayurvedic text said to be written in 1000 BC.
Ahita	Unhappy, miserable
Akasha	Ether, one of the five elements, also sky.
Ama	A substance which accumulates in the joints due to improper digestion and causes rheumatism.
Amavata	Rheumatism
Anandamaya	One of the five layers which make up the individual, this helps in experiencing bliss.
Anantavata	Migraine
Annamaya	The physical body, one of the five layers of the individual.
Anumana	Inference, deduction
Artha	Wealth
Ashtasthana Pariksha	Eight-fold method of medical examination used by Ayurvedic physicians.
Asthi	Bone tissue
Astika Darshana	Branch of Indian philosophy which recognizes the authority of the Vedas.
Atharva	One of the four Vedic texts.
Atman	The soul, considered indestructible in Hindu philosophy.
Atreya	Ancient Hindu sage, one of the founding fathers of Ayurveda.
Ayur	Life
Bharadvaja	Ancient Hindu sage, one of the founders of Ayurveda.
Brahma	The Creator, one of the gods of the Hindu holy trinity. The other two are Shiva, the Destructor and Vishnu, the Preserver.

Brahmans	Amongst Hindus, the class which by convention is supposed to comprise the educated priests.
Brimhana	Nourishing therapy usually prescribed for old, emaciated and weak people. One of the six basic Ayurvedic therapies.
Chapati	Small round cakes of coarse, unleavened bread eaten as an accompaniment in most Indian meals.
Charaka	Ancient Hindu sage who wrote the most authoritative Ayurvedic text *Charaka Samhita* based on the *Agnivesha Samhita.*
Daksha Prajapati	According to Hindu legend, Brahma's son.
Darshana	General term for systems of Indian philosophy, also means visual observation in Ayurvedic diagnosis.
Dhanwantari	The Hindu god of medicine.
Dhara	Therapy involving the use of medicated oils.
Dharma	In Hindu philosophy an individual's role and duties in life, decided by his birth, class and occupation.
Dhatus	Tissue elements.
Dinacharya	Regimen prescribed by Ayurveda to be followed during the day to prevent diseases.
Doshas	Basic functional units of the body. There are three, according to Ayurveda.
Ghee	A type of clarified liquid butter used widely in India both as a cooking base and for general consumption.
Gridhrasi	Sciatica
Griva Sandhigata Vata	Cervical Spondylosis.
Gunas	Basic attributes which characterize
Hikkaroga	physical and psychological reality. There are three in all—*sattva, rajas, tamas.* An attack of hiccups.
Hita	Happy, good
Homa	The act of offering oblations like pouring clarified butter into a sacred fire, an important ritual in Hindu worship.
Hridroga	Heart disease
Jala	Water, one of the five elements.
Jwara	Fever
Kalpa	Literally, art. In this case, therapy.
Kama	Desire for love and sex.
Kamala	Jaundice
Kapha	Phlegm, if roughly translated. According to Ayurveda, one of the three doshas or basic units of the body.
Kaphaja	That which originates from kapha.
Kasa Roga	Bronchitis
Kashyapa	One of the founding sages of Ayurveda.
Koshas	Successive layers which make up the individual.
Krimija	Heart disease caused due to external organisms which enter the body.
Langhana	Lightening therapy which helps remove unwanted and poisonous matter from the body through enema, emesis, control of thirst etc. One of the six basic Ayurvedic therapies.
Madhumeha	Diabetes
Mahabhuta	The basic elements which make up the universe. There are five in all—earth, water, fire, ether, air.
Majja	Bone marrow
Malas	Human waste products which include stool, urine, perspiration, ear wax, saliva.
Mamsa	Muscle tissue
Manomaya	One of the five layers that make up the

	individual; the psyche or what the individual thinks.
Marga	Route, way
Medas	Fat
Medoroga	Obesity
Moksha	Ultimate salvation in Hindu philosophy which signifies freedom from the ceaseless cycle of birth and death.
Nadi pariksha	Pulse examination.
Nastika Darshana	Branch of Indian philosophy which does not acknowledge the authority of the Vedas.
Nidana	Causes of a disease.
Ojas	A substance formed during the metabolic transformation of tissue elements which is vital to the individual's survival as it provides immunity.
Paittika	That which originates from pitta.
Pancha Mahabhuta	The five elements.
Parashara	One of the ancient founding sages of Ayurveda.
Pariksha	Examination
Pitta	One of the doshas. If loosely translated, it is bile.
Prakriti	Physical and psychological constitution of an individual.
Pranamaya	One of the five layers which make up the individual, it is the layer which enables an individual to feel and experience.
Prashna	To question or interrogate.
Pratyaksha	Form of Ayurvedic examination in which the physician directly relies on his five senses: seeing, hearing, smelling, touching and tasting, to diagnose a patient.
Pravahika	Amoebic dysentery.
Prithvi	Earth, one of the five elements.
Purvarupa	The premonitory symptoms of a disease.
Rajas	One of the three attributes of physical and psychological reality, *rajas* symbolises energy and passion.
Rakta	The red fraction of the blood.
Rasa	The remaining part of blood which contains the plasma after the red blood cells have been separated.
Rasayana	A therapy of rejuvenation which aims at reducing the effects of ageing.
Rasona kalpa	An intense and complex kind of rejuvenation therapy involving the use of garlic.
Ratricharya	Regimen prescribed by Ayurveda to be followed through the night to prevent diseases.
Rig	One of the four Vedic texts.
Rupa	The actual symptoms of a disease.
Sama	One of the four Vedic texts, also a state of perfect health when all the three doshas are equally balanced in the body.
Samprapti	The way a disease is finally manifested in the body.
Sanchara marga	The path of transportation of a disease.
Sannipata	The state in which all three doshas are imbalanced and the body is in imperfect health.
Sattva	One of the three attributes of reality, *sattva* signifies consciousness.
Shabda	Already existing statements about a disease made by experts based on their research.
Shuta	Colic pain
Snehana	Oleation therapy, also one of the six

83

	basic therapies. In this oil, *ghee* and even bone marrow is used.
Sparshana	To touch
Srota	Channels of circulation which carry external nutrient matter to the body organs and remove metabolic waste.
Stambhana	This is an astringent therapy which checks excessive physiological secretions.
Sthana	Place
Sushruta	One of the founding sages of Ayurveda, he wrote the famous Ayurvedic text *Sushruta Samhita*.
Swedana	One of the six basic therapies of Ayurveda, this involves fomentation.
Taila	Oil
Tamaka swasa	Bronchial asthma
Tamas	One of the three basic attributes of reality, *tamas* signifies mass and stability.
Udbhava sthana	Site of origination of a disease.
Unani tibb	Graeco-Arabic medicine. This originated in ancient Greece and was expanded upon in the Arabian world between the 8th and the 13th centuries.
Unmada	Hysteria
Upasaya	An initial method to explore the nature of a disease, keeping in mind the symptoms and looking for possible diagnoses.
Vata	One of the three doshas or basic functional units of the body. Loosely translated, it is wind.
Vata slaishmika jwara	Influenza
Vatika	That which originates from vayu or vata.
Vayu	Same as vata.
Veda	Ancient Aryan texts which contain the kernel of Indian philosophy, religious practises, customs, modes of living etc. There are four Vedic texts—*Rig, Yajur, Sama, Atharva*. These texts were compiled in a written form by disciples of Hindu sages from centuries of knowledge passed down orally. They are not the work of a single person.
Vichachika	Eczema
Vijnanmaya	One of the layers that make up the individual, it signifies the intellect which can discriminate between base and pure, right and wrong.
Yajur	One of the four Vedic texts.
Yoga	A form of physical exercise requiring extreme mental concentration which according to Indian philosophy, elevates the mind to a spiritual plane, thereby satisfying the demands of the body-mind-spirit complex.